PRAISE FOR
Caring, The Human Mode of Being

"*Caring, The Human Mode of Being* is a profoundly inspiring, intimate and authentic exploration of the author's understanding of human caring. It entices readers to reflect on who we are as persons, as family, as community; what it means to care; why we are in health service; and why we should move beyond our professional roles to understand human caring in relation to 'being-in-the-world.' It affirms that human caring is alive today in health care, despite the reality of limited resources, increasing workloads, restructuring and downsizing. It beautifully illuminates the forces of the human spirit that are triumphing today amidst the chaos in health care. Because of this, it is a **must read** for those of us who care about the future of our health care system.

"The book has broad interdisciplinary appeal and is recommended reading for all professionals who are part of a community of persons who provide service to others. It raises challenging issues for educators, practitioners and researchers about how we prepare and become professionally caring persons, and how we shape practice, research and educational environments to allow caring to happen.

"This work, however, moves beyond the boundaries of the health professions and challenges contemporary readers to consider their responsibilities for caring in relation to the universe. The author presents a compelling call to each of us as individuals and professionals to do something to demonstrate that caring is indeed the human mode of being. Having read the book, it will be difficult for anyone to ignore the call."

Angela Gillis, RN, PhD, Professor and Chair
Department of Nursing
St. Francis Xavier University
Antigonish, Nova Scotia

"Nursing is the most complex and demanding of all the health disciplines and, paradoxically, the least understood. Simone Roach writes about nursing in a way that can be understood by nurses and by non-nurses alike. In this second revision of her book, *Caring, The Human Mode of Being*, she presents some challenging thoughts and ideas borne of her consideration of new developments in postmodern philosophy, theology, physics and technology. At a time when 'caring' seems to have fallen off the political and health services' agendas, this book speaks to many nurses who struggle to care for people in societies where the human mode of being is no longer understood."

Dr. Elizabeth S. Farmer
Department of Nursing and Midwifery
University of Sterling
Inverness, Scotland

"In her work, Sister Simone calls us to understand who we are as human persons and our oneness with God and His universe. Her extraordinary synthesis and integration of understandings and experiences frame the exquisite view she casts on the sacredness and value of human life. Her work emanates from her soul and may well be called 'hallowed' and she a 'sage'."

Anne Boykin, RN, PhD, Dean
College of Nursing
Florida Atlantic University
Boca Raton, Florida

"Relevant, sound and well-grounded. Written with such a spirit of care. Engaging, inviting the reader to reflection. The SIX Cs apply to all. Delightfully Canadian with a universal theme."

Margaret Brennan, IHM, Professor Emerita
Regis College
University of Toronto
Toronto, Ontario

"With gifts of theological insight and poetic expression, Simone Roach offers a deeply inspirational work which shows the art of nursing and other forms of professional caring to be an expression of our deepest goodness as ethical beings."

Stan van Hooft, Associate Professor
School of Social Inquiry—Philosophical Studies
Faculty of Arts
Deakin University
Burwood, Australia

"This book offers a rare insight into a human phenomenon—caring—which we often assume we know well. The wealth of reflection on a wide variety of experiences of caring, and philosophical and theological thought on the matter, reveals clearly how much more we need to delve into this subject. The book can be profitably used by students, health care professionals, people engaged in ministry—indeed by any who are committed to caring."

Ronald A. Mercier, SJ, Vice-President and Dean
Regis College
University of Toronto
Toronto, Ontario

Caring, The Human Mode of Being

A Blueprint for the Health Professions

Second Revised Edition

M. Simone Roach, CSM

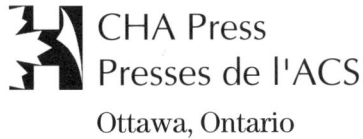
CHA Press
Presses de l'ACS
Ottawa, Ontario

Published by CHA Press, 17 York Street, Ottawa, ON K1N 9J6
Tel. (613) 241-8005; Fax (613) 241-5055, chapress@cha.ca
© 1987, 2002 by Sister M. Simone Roach. All rights reserved.
First Edition published in 1987. Second Revised Edition 2002. Reprinted 2004.

National Library of Canada Cataloguing in Publication Data

Roach, M. Simone (Marie Simone), 1922–
    Caring, the human mode of being : a blueprint for the health professions

2nd rev. ed.
Includes bibliographical references and index.
ISBN 1-896151-44-2

    1. Nursing—Philosophy.   2. Nursing ethics. I. Title.
RT84.5.R63 20021   610.73'01   C2002-900707-0

The use of any part of this publication, reproduced, stored in a retrieval system, or transmitted in any form or by any means, electronic, mechanical, photocopying, recording, or otherwise, without the prior written permission of the publisher and author — or, in the case of photocopying or other reprographic copying, a license from the Canadian Copyright Licensing Agency (CANCOPY) — is an infringement of the copyright law.

PRINTED IN CANADA
   3 5 4 2

*To all who, through
the goodness of others, continue to develop
their capacity to care and who personally and
professionally reverence the holy in all
of creation.*

CONTENTS

FOREWORD	vii
ACKNOWLEDGMENTS	ix
PROLOGUE	1

1. A CONTEXT — 7
- The Universe: Subject and Object of Care — 13
- Human Suffering: Problem or Mystery — 14
- Person and Technology: The Technological Imperative — 15
- Need for an Intelligent, Responsible Approach — 21

2. CARING, THE HUMAN MODE OF BEING — 23
- Why Is Reflection on Human Caring Important? — 27
- A Conceptualization — 38

3. REFLECTIONS ON CARING ATTRIBUTES — 41
- The Caring Universe — 41
- The SIX Cs — 43
- A Further Elaboration of the SIX Cs — 50
- Summary — 66

4. CARING AND PROFESSIONAL ETHICS — 67
- Introduction: Understanding the Language — 69
- Caring, Ethics and the Moral Life — 70
- Summary — 81

5. PROFESSIONS, PROFESSIONALISM AND TRUST — 83
- Trust and Boundary Violations — 87
- How the Health Care System Structures the Workplace — 90

Contents

    The Call of Care   93
    Summary   97

6. Healing through Story   99
    The Universe Story   103
    "The Cosmic Walk"   111

7. Education and Practice for Professional Caring   117
    Education and Practice as Transformative   117
    Health Services in a Historical Context   120
    Transformative Learning: A Global Perspective   122
    Transformative Learning: Caring as Response to Value   124
    Affective Response and "Being Affected"   128
    Transformative Learning: Caring as Virtuous Actions   130
    Transformative Learning: Practice of SIX Cs   131
    Transformative Learning: Reflective and Contemplative Practice   133
    Summary   137

Epilogue   139

Bibliography   145

Index   159

FOREWORD

Caring, The Human Mode of Being begins with a spirituality of vision into the worth of human life. Its author, M. Simone Roach, CSM, is able to articulate from the outset a sense of spiritual awe before the other as in God's image. The other is discovered as deeply worthy, not because of personal achievements, social usefulness, appearance or any other mundane measure, but simply because of inherent universal dignity under a sacred protective canopy. The human self is related to a presence in the universe greater than its own, and from this beginning point flow both right relations between persons and with the environment, both earthly and cosmic.

One of the most useful themes throughout this book is that the respect for life and environment, which contrasts with violence and underlies all caring motivations, is sustained by a sense of divine creativity. The religious language of unlimited *love* is resonant with the contemporary ethics of *care*, and these two terms are used throughout in a creative dialogue. "The fundamental thesis of this work is that caring is the human mode of being," the author writes, despite the reality of encounters with evil even in its more demonic forms such as genocide.

Caring is definitive of nursing, and the author's careful discussion of the clinical context from her perspective as a nurse is compelling. Other chapters address care for the environment and for the universe that sustains it. The book ends with a powerful note—education in ethics does not necessarily touch students deeply enough to enable them to become more caring people. The discussion of various clinical quandaries and moral dilemmas—however interesting—is not in itself *transformative* learning which results in virtuous action. It is toward such transformative learning that ethics education must now move.

This is a creative and serious book, one that brings together the virtue of care with a spirituality of the worth of human life, nature and the wonder of our universe. It is ultimately quite practical in presenting a pedagogy of transformation that merits our considered attention. Sister M. Simone Roach has created a splendid book that will be of great interest to a wide audience of persons asking the question, *Whatever happened to care?* Care can be recovered despite pressures to limit its compass. But such recovery may require the fuller spiritual vision available to human nature in its fullness.

Stephen G. Post, PhD
Center for Biomedical Ethics
School of Medicine
Case Western Reserve University

ACKNOWLEDGMENTS

This book was written by many people, beginning in my family, where the Christian faith was nurtured and where reaching out to others, sharing the little we had, was a way of life. A wonderful high school English teacher, Sister Cecilia Lawrence, a Sister of Charity of Halifax, called forth a life-interest in writing. The Sisters of St. Martha of Antigonish shaped the beginning of my nursing career and, later, as a member of the Martha Community, they provided me with the educational and professional opportunities that fostered my development in nursing education and research. This work is really theirs and would not have been possible without their support and prayer.

Formal writing on human caring began in 1984 with the publication of *Caring: The Human Mode of Being, Implications for Nursing*, the first in a monograph series under the leadership of Kathleen Arpin, Faculty of Nursing, University of Toronto. For many years prior to this publication, the University of Toronto had a formative influence on my vision of nursing education and practice. One need only recall the names of Kathleen Russell, Nettie Douglas Fidler, Florence Emory and their many successors to realize the impact of its leadership in Canada and elsewhere. This vision continues to be inspired and challenged by my association with the International Association for Human Caring.

A year as visiting scholar at Regis College offered the time, space and access to limitless resources at the University of Toronto. I am deeply grateful to Ronald A. Mercier, SJ, dean and vice-president, who made this possible, and for his availability and generous consultation despite administrative, teaching and other commitments. Lorna Young, head librarian at Regis was always available and Barbara Geiger, reference librarian, in her efficiency in tracking sources, expedited my work on many occasions. The Sisters at St. Joseph's House of Studies, nourishing body, mind and spirit, helped me recoup the energy to meet the seemingly endless challenges of reading, computing and revising.

Acknowledgments

A casual meeting with Edmund O'Sullivan, the coordinator of the Transformative Learning Center at OISE, turned out to be a graced acquaintance. Through personal inspiration and his writings, Dr. O'Sullivan influenced the shape of this work. Stephen Dunn, the director of the Elliot Allen Institute of Theology and Ecology, St. Michael's University, contributed to my research by expanding my awareness of the global call for human care and by facilitating access to relevant personal and material resources.

The writings of Dr. Stephen Post, Center for Biomedical Ethics, Case Western Reserve University, inspire many, and I know his association with this work will enhance its quality and credibility. I am extremely grateful to him for so graciously consenting to write the Foreword.

This revised edition also includes several poems or verses from poems. I am grateful to the authors and to their publishers for allowing me to reprint them in this text.

- Mary Lou Kownacki and her publisher, Benetvision Press, for "The Blue Heron and Thirty-Seven Other Miracles" in the Prologue;
- Mary Elizabeth O'Brien and her publisher, Jones and Bartlett Publishers, for the poem from *Spirituality in Nursing: Standing on Holy Ground* at the end of the Prologue;
- Edwina Gateley and her publisher, Source Books, for "The Sharing" appearing at the beginning of chapter 6; and
- Katie Eriksson and her publisher, Almqvist and Wiksell, for "Reflections on Suffering" at the end of the Epilogue.

Acknowledgment for "The Cosmic Walk," cited in chapter 6, is given to Sister Miriam MacGillis, Genesis Farm, New Jersey, who conducted several workshops with the Sisters of St. Martha in Antigonish, Nova Scotia, and Lethbridge, Alberta, in April 1998.

Since the early 1980s, when the first edition of this book was conceived, Eleanor Sawyer, director of publishing, Canadian Healthcare Association Press, has been companion and advisor. Thank you, Eleanor, and gratitude also to all at CHA who once again bring to life a new publication.

PROLOGUE

At dawn
in late September
I sit on the deck
facing the fog
that engulfs Lake Findley,
close my eyes,
finger my beads,
and repeat slowly,
Sanctus, Sanctus, Sanctus.
Only the silent fog.
Nothing but silent fog.
Sanctus, Sanctus, Sanctus.
My eyes open.
The sun
has sliced a path
to the small island,
just beyond the shore.
A blue heron stares back.
Is this not a miracle?

(Mary Lou Kownacki, "Poem One")

In an age when chaos is the name for transition and change, when violence is all around us and uncertainty crafts the map of the future, we look for signs of hope for better things to come, for something to celebrate. Often we desire an extraordinary revelation, something beyond everyday experience to show all is right with our world. When we do not find what we are looking for, or even do not know the nature of the search itself, we have difficulty in continuing to fan the flame of expectancy. We are often slow to discover the real miracles that happen before our eyes. Mary Lou Kownacki (1996) shares her way of discovering the miraculous in *The Blue Heron and Thirty-Seven Other Miracles*. She suggests we "[t]ry to imagine how different life would be if we all recognized and reveled in the present, in the common, as sacrament" (7).

Sacrament, an encounter, a life ritual is a sacred sign and instrument of the holy. Sacraments are described as "the masterworks of God in the new and everlasting covenant" (Canadian Conference of Catholic Bishops 1994). In faith traditions, they are rituals of healing, involving the family and the community gathered around the person who is suffering, wounded or approaching death. Sacraments of healing take place in a sacred space—the space of health service—where both the sick and the caregiver enter into a bond of care. This bond of care is not unilateral; each person participates in a relationship that nourishes both the server and the one being served.

Health care is a moral enterprise. It is a moral enterprise because it establishes relationships with moral bonds involving duties and responsibilities. In any relationship, the need for trust in the worth and the inviolability of each person presupposes respect for human dignity. Such presupposition of respect not only applies to patient-client and family but also assumes the respect merited by the trustworthiness of the caregiver.

The relationship of persons in health service—doctors, nurses, therapists, clergy, pastoral care staff and others caring for patients—is a sacred one, since it involves entering into the lives of others with a degree of intimacy that is unique and bounded by special canons of loyalty. It is an encounter with patients, family members and significant others during times of crisis, need and dependency, with the expectation that each is *sacrament* for the other. It is a fragile relationship characterized by vulnerability on the side of the recipient, sometimes flawed by power explicitly or implicitly exercised by the caregiver.

The law recognizes the dignity of persons and provides for protection of privacy and for an individual's right to nonviolation of body, mind and spirit. Established legal boundaries guard the person's right to self-determination and provide strict protocols for consent and other procedures. And the law itself, delegated by common agreement to preserve the individual and common good, represents a public recognition of the moral sphere of human life and community. It is even made explicit in policies regarding care of the body after death. In this latter case, it is interesting to review how protocols for treating the body, donated for science after death, incorporate standards for respect not only in dissection and anatomical study but also in the prescriptions for burial.

It is not difficult to see how trespassing human boundaries of persons and families can be an affront to human dignity, and why in health care even the simple act of touching, if not consented to, can be a moral-legal violation. The termination of the life of a human being, the growing acceptance of feticide, violations such as rape, which attack the inner sanctuary of the person and kill the soul, and practices that isolate human beings to the margins of society in poverty and desperation or as political outcasts are moral outrages—sins of humanity. These outrages not only affect the individual on whom they are inflicted, but also dehumanize society as communal and collective, diminishing the lustre of its moral fiber. Human beings have been created by love, for love, to love.

This work is focused on caring as the human mode of being, with reflections on what it means to be a human person, and on the canons of respect for human dignity which are the guardians of both personhood and community. Caring is grounded in an attitude of *religio* before all creation and is a reminder to human beings of who they are in a manner never before comprehended. As creatures of a universe become more visible in its network of interconnectedness, human beings have the capacity and the call to be sacred signs, to be sacrament within all of creation.

Threaded through the reflections of this work are questions, hopefully not interpreted as judgmental or acrimonious. These reflective questions are simply intended to convey an openness to explore the mystery of our lives, the miracles all around us, the preciousness of human life and that of all otherkind. They are intended to accent the call of care as expressive of professional identity, of moral agency at a time in our world when the values of the marketplace take priority over personal and common good. And as persons whose professional identity is to care, these reflections have served to remind the writer, and hopefully will engage the reader in contemplating the global parameters, of responsibility and accountability. Each day we are confronted with the reality of what, as family and global community, we have done and are doing to life on this planet. It is a time to celebrate but also a time to mourn.

Human care is presented as virtuous activity, and persons in health professions, by the very nature of their roles, are involved in acts shaped by natural and supernatural virtues. Caring is made real in the virtuous acts of caregivers as individuals, not dichotomized by personal-private, professional-public, practitioners-moral agents, but by persons who aspire to fulfillment of self through care of self and others.

It would be irresponsible to assert that this is, in fact, the way it is within all health care facilities and within the health system at large. Everything is not well within our health care system. The availability and quality of health services vary widely across the globe. And within so-called highly developed countries there are situations of which we cannot be proud. Sad commentaries on the quality of care are made with increasing frequency by family members who are distraught and frustrated because a loved one does not receive essential care, or because the care given sometimes causes more problems than it prevents. The frustration is borne equally by responsible, committed educators and practitioners who devote all their energy to transforming bad situations into possibilities for good. The *system* itself bears the brunt of the negative appraisals of health care, while at the same time, education models are revamped and reformed with the expectation that practitioners will be better able to be moral agents of change.

It is a difficult time to be in health care, a time of enormous challenge for caregivers, as well as for patients and families. But many good things are happening, and most people in human services want to do a good job. This work attempts to balance the negative with a firm belief and faith in the commitment of persons in health care management, policy, research, teaching and practice to a high quality of service.

It is said of our society that we have lost a sense of the sacred. But we see and experience the sacred in our personal, family and professional lives. The smile of a newborn baby, the beauty of a sunset or a double rainbow, the new buds struggling to come forth from the trees, the gorgeous birds returning from their stay in the south, the mounds of snow and even the burst of thunder and the lightening that illuminates the dark night all fascinate us. Perhaps we simply need to recover our sense of awe for the things we see and do everyday.

Mary Elizabeth O'Brien, in an opening reflection in her work on *Spirituality in Nursing: Standing on Holy Ground* (1999), provides a fitting conclusion to this prologue and sets a tone for the context of *Caring, The Human Mode of Being*. While the poem is referenced in nursing, it applies to all as human persons. I would suggest each individual reading this book—whether or not in a formal health care role—reflect on the occasions during a given day when an encounter with self or another person is an entry into and an experience of "Holy Ground."

> The nurse's smile warmly embraces the cancer patient arriving for a chemotherapy treatment.
> This is holy ground.
>
> The nurse watches solicitously over the pre-op child who tearfully whispers "I'm scared."
> This is Holy Ground.
>
> The nurse gently diffuses the anxieties of the ventilator-dependent patient in the ICU.
> This is Holy Ground.
>
> The nurse listens with a caring heart to the pain of the Alzheimer patient's loneliness.
> This is Holy Ground.
>
> The nurse lovingly sings hymns to the anencephalic infant dying in the nurse's arms.
> This is Holy Ground.

The nurse slips a comforting arm around the trembling shoulders of the newly bereaved widow.
    This is Holy Ground.

The nurse tenderly takes the hand of the frail elder struggling to accept life in the nursing home.
    This is Holy Ground.

The nurse
    reverently touches and is touched by
        the patient's heart,
            the dwelling place of the living God.

This is spirituality in nursing [in health care],
    this is the ground of the practice of nursing [of human encounter],
        this is holy ground!

            (Mary Elizabeth O'Brien, *Spirituality in Nursing*)

1

A CONTEXT

This book is about human caring, caring as the human mode of being. It is about caring for others and caring for self, about self-fulfillment and self-integration, and about the self transformed toward mature personhood. Human caring is about loving. Human beings are created by love, for love and bonded in a self-creating universe, energized and *fired* by love (Swimme and Berry 1992).

Authentic human caring is not subservience, not subordination, not subjection to control but a way of living that fosters human freedom in all relationships. It is not characterized by being excessively submissive but by being servant in relationship of covenant. For this reason, it is important to extricate an understanding of caring from a false identification with servitude and subjection, and from any bondage that gets in the way of personal freedom and professional relationships. Professional caring practice does not equal subservience.

This work is about human caring, grounded in our beliefs and perceptions about what it means to be a human person, a person wonderfully made in God's image—image, similitude and likeness. In all faith traditions there is recognition of a sacred bond between human beings and the *ultimate other*. In the Judeo-Christian creation story, after the *let there be* light, water, land, vegetation and all other living creatures, "God created man [the human being] in his image: in the divine image he created him; male and female he created them" (Gen. 1:27. For commentary, *see* Gula 1989, 64–74; Bruteau 1997).

The Creation Story is a story of gratuitous love. In the context of this story and the *new story* so wondrously revealed in science and cosmology, this biblical image provides inspiration and meaning for us in this postmodern age when human identity is such a central preoccupation. The thoughts of St. Irenaeus (circa 165–200) add to the celebratory vision of the preceding in his proclamation, *the glory of God is the human person fully alive; and the life of the human person is the vision of God*. As created in God's image, each person is sacred and gifted with a dignity that is, prior to any benefits of lineage or personal achievements, a perspective which is an antidote to the modern fixation on nonrelational individualism and a powerful model for all involved in human services.

The human person is not amenable to definition. An individual can be classified according to race, gender, religion, ethnicity and social class, but being a person transcends all descriptive categories. To be a person is to be who I am. It is to intuit at the core of one's being a "mystery which may be alluded to but never stated" (Feldstein 1978, 23), to ask the question not of *what* but of *who* (Heschel 1965), to embrace the project of human flourishing (Cahill 1996) and to understand more fully the meaning of the good life (Gula 1999). As human persons, we most frequently search for self-understanding in darkness and ambiguity and, in the words of Paul Tournier, "I can speak endlessly of myself to myself or to someone else, without ever succeeding in giving a complete and truthful picture of myself. There remains in every man [woman], even for himself [herself], something of impenetrable mystery" (1957, 13).

To be a person is always to be in relationship, to live in a community of persons, to seek for a community embraced by love. As noted previously, the human person is created from love, for love, to be love. Ronald Rolheiser (1999), introducing his work, *The Holy Longing*, paraphrases a quotation attributed to Plato: "We are fired into life with a madness that comes from the gods and which would have us believe that we can have a great love, perpetuate our own seed, and contemplate the divine" (3).

The metaphor, *madly in love*, is an apt qualifier for that experience of "an unquenchable fire, a restlessness, a longing, a disquiet, a hunger, a loneliness, a gnawing nostalgia, a wildness that cannot be tamed, a congenital all-embracing ache that lies at the center of human experience and is the ultimate force that drives everything else" (4). Rolheiser speaks of what we do with this fire inside us as a way of expressing our spirituality and reflects on our relationship with God, with others and with the cosmic world.

Finley (1978) refers to the spirituality of Thomas Merton as pivoting on the question of ultimate human identity. He discusses the lifelong challenge of the tension between the true and the false self noting "the core of our being is drawn like a stone to the quiet depths of each moment where God waits for us with eternal longing. But to those depths the false self will not let us travel" (26).

In understanding spirituality as derivative and expressive of ultimate human identity, it is helpful to make a distinction between spirituality, religion and theology. Sandra Schneiders (1999), in a three-part presentation, notes the confusion in contemporary use of these terms represented by comments such as " '[s]pirituality is very important to me but I am not interested in religion' " (Part 1, on-line). While she addresses such confusion, she notes they are closely related and mutually implicating.

Examining spirituality as life project and practice, Schneiders defines spirituality as " 'the experience of conscious involvement in the project of life-integration through self-transcendence toward the ultimate value one perceives' " (Ibid.). On the other hand, she notes, "[w]hat seems to mark religions is that they are cultural systems for dealing with ultimate reality, whether or not that ultimate reality is God, and they are institutionalized in patterns of creed, code and cult" (Part 2). Even within specific faith traditions, these cultural and institutional practices of religion vary greatly. Theology deals with beliefs in which an explicit faith is formulated and may be simply defined as " 'faith seeking understanding' " (Ibid., Part 3).

Specific faith traditions structure the manner in which participants within these traditions express their spirituality. The Christian thinks about spirituality as a striving for a more intimate union with God through Jesus Christ. Persons of the Jewish, Islamic and other faith traditions express spirituality in a different manner. Donal Dorr (1990), addressing a holistic spirituality, captures its personal, interpersonal and public aspects within a text from the prophet Micah:

> "You have been told. . . what is good, and what the Lord requires of you: Only to do right and to love goodness, and to walk humbly with your God" (6:8).

Other translations use language perhaps more familiar: *Act justly. Love tenderly. Walk humbly before your God*, clearly not pointing to a me and God spirituality but one immersed in relationships with people.

The relevance of the preceding reflections is significant, first, as a help to understanding our life project of human caring. What is the *stone* that draws us, the inner force that energizes us in our personal and professional lives? How does the call to live justly, love tenderly and walk humbly before our God shape personal life and professional practice? Why do individuals choose a particular profession in the first place? Second, in the care of patients-families, as well as in relationships with those with whom we work, the preceding reflections hopefully serve as a helpful reminder of the need to respect individual differences. Madeleine Leininger, in her life work on cultural care diversity and universality, provides a model for health care that integrates these cultural understandings.

As much as we may theorize about love as eros, as filia, as agape, theorizing in itself does not adequately capture the inner aspirations of all persons whose *holy longing* is to love and be loved, unless it is tied to the experience of loving and being loved. Such experience is rooted in the unique journey of each person, confirmed in relationships, and shaped by personal choice or lack of it. What is done with this desire to love and be loved reflects how one's values are integrated within a way of being with God, with self and with others. Application of this insight in ministry in the service professions can lead to a more attentive engagement of self in identification of needs and provision of care.

The desire to love and be loved is at the heart of the human condition, at the root of human searching and a prevailing undercurrent so easily missed in the needs of persons suffering from illness, disease and disability. In everyday encounters, the caregiver meets human persons who *happen to be* patients-clients, family members, colleagues and staff. It may be helpful to ask, How does attunement to this realization of the lovableness and the need for love of each human being, even with appropriate *professional distance*, structure the health care environment and professional relationships? Each human person is beloved because he or she is the beloved of God (Nouwen 1992). Care as the precondition for all cure assimilates this and involves a great deal more than expert knowledge and competent technology.

Stephen Post (1990) reflects on agape as an "affection of the heart, an attunement of the person's deepest center that issues in a faithful will to exist for God and others as well as for one's own true fulfillment" (116). Post's reflections do not come from what he calls a superficial universalism but from an understanding of agape, "grounded in narrative and sustained and reinforced in religious fellowship by reliable acts of reciprocation. It is a narrative reinforcing through story, response and affirmation our existing for others" (90).

In his 1994 work, *Spheres of Love*, Post discusses love in special relations, especially marriage and familial ties. But he also considers how love for those near and dear in filial relationships can be, needs to be, balanced with love for the stranger—the neighbor.

Challenging the *whatever the user wishes* meaning of love, he provides the following inclusive overview:

> Love is manifested in solicitude (anxious concern) for the welfare of self and others, and usually in a delight in the presence of the other. Love is an abrogation of the self-centered tendency—although not of all concern for the self—and a transfer of interests to the other for his or her own sake on the basis of the other's existence alone, his or her positive properties, or a combination of both. Love is the foundation of all moral idealism, i.e. of acts that surpass the minimal requirements of "do no harm". . . . But love goes beyond prudential moral minimalism because it represents a shift of the self toward actions for the good of others, and is a much more exacting standard than "do no harm." Love requires the acceptance of a self-sacrifice justly limited by reasonable degrees of self-concern, lest love become oppressive and destructive of the agent (4–5).

In their work titled, *The Crisis of Care*, Phillips and Benner (1994) echo Post's position, noting the importance of discovering caring where it is evident in practice, and nurturing and restoring caring practice through narrative.

The human person is also a sexual being, experiencing self as male or female in relationship to self and others. Sexuality draws individuals out of themselves into relationships with others, seeking communion and wholeness. It is again an expression of that energy that strives for communion, community and friendship. Speaking of sexual difference and parenthood, Lisa Cahill refers to gender as a *moral* project that entails

> the social humanization of biological tendencies, capacities, and differences, including the social ties that they, by their very nature, are inclined to create. Biological sex differences and male and female parenthood—both the sexual cooperation it necessitates and the social partnership it sponsors—are more opportunity than limit. They provide a ground and content for the human virtues of love, commitment, respect, equality, and the building of social unity toward the common good (1996, 89).

Nonetheless, in saying this, Cahill also recognizes the perversion of these relationships in situations of domination, infidelity and objectification.

In an article by Selling, the human person adequately considered stands in relation to everything, to the whole of reality, to the material world. The person is cultural, always in relation to groups of other persons, and historical, deriving their meaning from the past and toward the future. Adequately considered, the human person stands in relation to and is mediated through other human beings—family, friends, teachers and mentors. But as Selling goes on to reflect, "[t]he 'person' is not simply a material, cultural, historical, social, relational entity but a 'self' " (1998, 105), called to freedom and responsibility. This freedom is not simply the ability to make choices but to experience one's personal identity, to experience a conscious interiority. It is reflected in the most secret and sacred core of the person—conscience. The human person adequately considered is a corporeal subject, a unique individual, a one-time occurrence (Ibid., 96–109). The parent, the caregiver, the patient, student or teacher is not just one among many, not just a daily statistic or a number on a time card. The danger of being caught in structures of bureaucracy is that it is perhaps easier to be a *cog in the wheel*; it requires more energy to invest in being a person.

To be a person is to be in relation both according to one's nature and vocation. It is the universal call of being in relation with all humankind and otherkind, of being in intimate connection with the universe through origin and evolution, through the past, the present and the future.

THE UNIVERSE: SUBJECT AND OBJECT OF CARE

To be persons of care is to recognize that our relationships go beyond the immediate claims of daily living. It is to situate ourselves within a wider universe dependent both on the application of science and technology for its discovery and celebration, and on the attentiveness of all human beings for its survival and sustainability. At this time, our relationship with the earth and with all of creation is not for us simply a matter to know *about*. It is rather a call to responsibility, a passionate appeal to comprehend in a manner that draws each person into an awareness of the fragility of all living systems, into a consciousness of an imminent crisis of planetary survival. It is human caring that evokes a sense of urgency for the preservation of every species on planet earth; that commits a person more fully to a call to life-giving, life-enhancing, life protection of human and otherkind.

Anne Lonergan and Carolyn Richards (1987) cite some of the important works that have addressed this relationship between human beings and the earth, and the planetary dimensions of the contemporary crisis, noting Gibson Winter 1981, James Gustafson 1982 and Jurgen Moltmann 1985. In *God in Creation: A New Theology of Creation and the Spirit of God,* Moltmann notes:

> What we call the environmental crisis is not merely a crisis in the natural environment of human beings. It is nothing less than a crisis in human beings themselves. It is a crisis of life on this planet, a crisis so comprehensive and so irreversible that it can not unjustly be described as apocalyptic. It is not a temporary crisis. As far as we can judge, it is the beginning of a life and death struggle for creation on this earth (xi).

Prophets of our time echo the works of Teilhard de Chardin (*The Divine Milieu*, 1960 and *The Phenomenon of Man*, 1959). Primary among these spokespersons is Thomas Berry, a cultural historian referred to as a *geologian*. *The Universe Story* (1992), coauthored with Brian Swimme, a mathematical cosmologist, has already become a classic work. This *new story*, the most exciting story of our time, can be viewed as a wake-up call to care. The following resources are but a limited selection of a continuously expanding literature in this field: Carson 1962, Berry 1988, Swimme 1988, Swimme and Berry 1992, Lonergan and Richards 1987, Conlon 1994, Scharper 1997, and Hessel and Ruether 2000. Opportunities for study in such areas as cosmology, ecology, eco-justice, ecotheology, ecophilosophy and ecofeminism have become available in recent years. The Elliot Allen Institute for Theology and Ecology at St. Michael's University, Toronto, is one example of a program of study in the disciplines of theology and ecology.

HUMAN SUFFERING: PROBLEM OR MYSTERY

Existentially, the human person is never in complete harmony with self, with others and with God. Each person is acquainted with infirmity, manifested in numerous ways in the woundedness of self and immediate others; knows physical, emotional and spiritual pain; and participates in human suffering personally and collectively. Human health, that dynamic state of ease, harmony and integration, is mirrored experientially in various degrees of its absence—in dis-ease, dis-harmony, dis-integration, shared by the whole human family. Persons dedicated to human service professions meet such everyday, for the health care world is "the meeting point of the anxieties and major questions now preoccupying humanity" (Tillard 1981, 17). For many people, suffering is considered within the *normal* expectations of an ordinary human life, remaining a mystery to be contemplated not a problem to be solved. But, for many, relief of suffering inspires the commitment of a lifetime; for others, suffering represents a basic evil to be overcome at any cost—even at the cost of human life itself.

History and everyday experience tell another story, an account of the inhumanity of human persons to brothers and sisters because of race, social class and ethnic backgrounds. Individuals and groups who attempt to intervene in matters of political corruption and injustice are imprisoned or, in some instances, not heard of anymore. Those who simply try to raise community consciousness about poverty and environmental issues are frequently suspect. It is not always easy to do good!

The twentieth century is viewed as the most violent in the history of humankind, a record about which all humanity needs to mourn. In the face of such evil, it is understandably difficult to believe that caring is the human mode of being. Nonetheless, the challenge of this work is to encourage reflection on hope and future promise; on the commitment of many ordinary people whose lives are characterized by fidelity and service to family and neighbor; on the goodness of human persons even when tested by rejection, poverty and gross dehumanization; on the perennial triumph of the human spirit.

PERSON AND TECHNOLOGY: THE TECHNOLOGICAL IMPERATIVE

This is a wonderfully graced time in which to live. But it is a critical point in time, fraught with new responsibilities never before encountered by humankind. Dr. Ursula Franklin, an experimental physicist and professor emeritus at the University of Toronto, notes the change in understanding technology, from the grounded practice of working and living together to a culture of compliance and the acceptance of external control and management. She observes:

> Today the values of technology have so permeated the public mind that all too frequently what is efficient is seen as the right thing to do. Conversely, when something is perceived to be wrong, it tends to be critiqued in practical terms as being inefficient, or counterproductive (a significant term in its own right). The public discourse I am urging here needs to break away from the technological mindset to focus on justice, fairness, and equality in the global sense. Once technological practices are questioned on a principled basis and, if necessary, rejected on that level, new practical ways of doing what needs to be done will evolve (1990, 123).

Health care, particularly in the Western world, has profited immensely by phenomenal developments in science and technology, and expertise has become the norm rather than the exception in the scientific community. As this work is in progress, the report of the International Genome Program, one of many spectacular revelations of the beginning of this twenty-first century, is being released. What will we do with the knowledge we acquire? Echoing Franklin's concern, the technological imperative, *what can be done ought to be done*, has never been such a threat, never so open to challenge. And the issues around what drives apparent success have never been so close to the edge of a moral quagmire.

The example of human cloning, which has moved quickly from scientific possibility to user-friendly technology, seems to be a final test of scientific responsibility and, therefore, credibility. If human life is nothing more than material and commodity, then *creation* and destruction become a logical consequence. If individuals and couples have a *right* to a child, and if this right is attended to by whatever means technologically possible, the dignity of individual personhood becomes a questionable value. Is human cloning motivated by human care, grounded in reverence for the sacredness of life, and respect for the noninstrumental dignity of the human person? Or is it essentially fired by ambition, vested interest, the hubris of some who, in the name of science, direct their knowledge and expertise for profit and in response to the pressures of the market? If (when) a *human being* is cloned, does the product become simply an artifact of biological engineering? If reverence for the sacredness of human life is replaced by the negotiable at any cost, if know-how replaces vision, then we have reason to fear that science as applied as technoscience has lost its soul.

In 1974, Hans Jonas, a prophet for our time, speaking of the inadequacy of the then prevailing ethic to provide dependable norms for personal and public behavior, noted: "[W]e shiver in the nakedness of a nihilism in which near-omnipotence is paired with near-emptiness, greatest capacity with least knowing what for" (17). He uses the implications of biological engineering as an example of complexity and ambiguity, particularly in the manner in which engineering itself has been understood. In the conventional sense, engineering meant the designing and constructing of material artifacts for human use. Technology has been concerned with lifeless materials. The advent of biological engineering, according to Jonas, "signals a radical departure from this clear division, indeed a break of metaphysical importance: Man [the human person] becomes the direct object as well as the subject of the engineering art" (142–143).

Jonas continues his reflection on the change in the conventional relation between mere experiment and real action. He notes "the experiment *is* the real deed, and the real deed *is* an experiment" (144). In mechanical construction, things are reversible: in human engineering, in engineering of all living beings—all with a code of genetic identity—deeds are irrevocable. For genetic engineering, Jonas asserts, mechanical engineering offers no analog. While developments in genetic engineering are a source of control over generation and heredity, provide hope for significant breakthroughs in the prevention of disorders of genetic origin and, with almost daily advances, bring new expectations for cure of certain diseases, is not Jonas' reminder still cogent for the twenty-first century?

Referring to what he calls the final triumph of power, he observes that it is a power which, once exercised, "is out of the wielder's hand, dispatched into the play of life's vaster complexity which defies complete analysis and prediction: on that count the power, however fateful, is blind" (145). In 1974, Jonas raised a perennial but radically cogent question that is unmistakably the question for our time: "We stumble into ultimate questions as soon as we propose to tamper with the making of man. They all converge into one: in what image?" (146). In biological engineering, in tampering with the creation of human life, are we becoming *sorcerer's apprentices*, setting in motion what we can neither control nor reverse?

At the time of this writing, the media covered daily reports on human cloning. A commentary by James Le Fanu (2000) on developments in legislation by the British Parliament echoes Jonas' concerns and that of many others. Speaking of the *scientific heavyweights* of the Royal Society, the Human Fertilization and Embryology Authority, the Human Genetics Commission and the Nuffield Council on Bioethics, he notes they arrived at a conclusion: "The potential therapeutic benefits are so great, there is no alternative—cloning must be legalized" (1,628). Le Fanu challenges the arguments presented by these groups in favor of cloning, points to the inaccuracy of their assumptions and notes other less invasive means for achieving the proposed, potential benefits.

In a special to the *Toronto Star* on 10 March 2001, the headline read: "Scientists set to clone first human." According to this report, the three members of the team—Dr. Severino Antinori of Italy, Dr. Panayiotis M. Zavos, an American reproductive physiologist, and Dr. Avi Ben-Abraham, an American-Israeli biotechnologist, told critics nothing can stop their plan to create cloned children, and they noted more than six hundred infertile couples had signed up for the program. According to the report, they spurned the idea of submitting to ethical or scientific oversight by any government. On the same day, the *National Post* also published a front-page story under the headline "Research Called 'Criminal'." In it, Michael Higgins, philosopher and ethicist, noted: "[N]ow that we have crossed into the third millenium, we have the technology to break the rules of nature." Dr. Margaret Somerville of McGill University Centre for Medicine, Ethics and Law is also quoted as saying, "This is the single greatest power we have had up to this point, the power to create life, and we are blithely going ahead. There is something to be said for not crossing these boundaries. Every human being has the right to be an individual and the right to be a surprise to themselves."

This one example of human cloning, reflecting an emerging societal ethos, is perhaps the most gargantuan issue facing the moral community at this time, and the questions, Ought it to be done because it can be? and In whose image? are paramount. Raising issues of concern here is not antiscience but refers rather to the importance of higher-order questions. What ought to be the moral-ethical ground rules around experimentation and tampering with human life? What is the basis for belief in the sacred, in the sanctity of human life, in the value of life in all otherkind? How do we recover what has been a traditional pillar of medical ethics: *First of all do no harm?* Commentaries continue to be presented in the media and complex issues heighten the controversy. A sobering question remains: Will wisdom and a vision of the sacred prevail over or shape the prevailing societal ethos? Will the prophets be heard? Albert Einstein made the following comment:

> Concern for man himself must always constitute the chief objective of all technological effort—concern for the big, unsolved problems of how to organize human work and the distribution of commodities in such a manner as to assure that the results of our scientific thinking may be a blessing to mankind, and not a curse (Circa 1930s).

Einstein is also remembered for asserting that we cannot simultaneously prevent and prepare for war.

How do we hallow the knowledge and expertise of eminent scientists, celebrate advances in science and technology, and honor progress and human flourishing out of a moral response of reverence, out of an attitude of *religio* and respect for all life on this planet? How do we integrate traditional wisdom with modern progress? Respect for human life has foundations in the natural awareness of the sacred in the customs of peoples, as well as being enshrined in faith traditions. In the following commentary, Shils throws light on the apprehension expressed by many at the present time about tampering with the creation of human life, seeing respect for life as arising out of something deep within the human psyche:

> The source of the revulsion or apprehension is deeper than the culture of Christianity and its doctrine of the soul. Indeed, it might be said that the Christian doctrine was enabled to maintain its long prosperity and to become so effective because it was able to conform for so many centuries to a deeper, protoreligious "natural metaphysic." Cultural traditions play a part in sustaining the sense of revulsion but they themselves would not go on if they were not continuously impelled by this "natural metaphysic" (1967, 41).

Lisa Cahill (1977) speaks to the foundation for respect for human life in natural law.

> Although religious belief in a Divine Maker Who loves and sustains personal life provides a strong warrant for respect, the principle of the sanctity of life can also be defended on philosophical grounds, by an appeal to common human experience. Many an atheistic or agnostic humanist would agree that since life is the fundamental and irreplaceable condition of the experience of all human values, it is a basic, or *the* basic, value and must not be destroyed without grave cause (48).

Our society is often accused of being nonreflective, and persons in service professions, often required to make life-dependent decisions on their feet, are at a high level of risk. As we contemplate who we are as human persons, immersed in personal, family and professional conflicts and challenges, caught in a paradigm of mechanistic thinking and wooed by technological breakthroughs and possibilities, the discernment of truth calls for great wisdom. Bound by restrictive structures in the workplace, pressures of zero-budget management and finding the ideals of caring challenged by the realities of the numbers of persons to be served, great moral support and stamina are required simply to hang in. Aware of living on a planet, where all living beings and supports for life are diminishing daily, and seeing that even a little *something* can be done demands faith. Perhaps the worst possible scenario for persons called to care is to bathe in the comfort and luxury of denial.

A religious fundamentalist might argue that God is going to come and take care of everything; destroy the perpetrators and save us who are guiltless! The real issue is that it is we who are doing ourselves in. If the planet is being destroyed, human beings are responsible. If, as the commentary by Higgins previously asserts, we use the technology we have to break the rules of nature, the resulting, unpredictable future, with its consequences for good or ill will, have to be borne by us and our descendants.

NEED FOR AN INTELLIGENT, RESPONSIBLE APPROACH

The transcendental method of Bernard Lonergan (1971) offers a pattern for guided thought and action that has universal application, in harmony with an orderly, objectified process of being attentive, intelligent, reasonable and responsible. This methodology calls for *attentiveness, experiencing the experience* of what is going on around us. This embraces the everyday experience of people on the streets in our cities and neighborhoods, in the culture of health care and related workplaces and in the political environment and its influence on national and international boundaries and lifestyles. It has to do with sensitization, for example, to daily reports on global climate change and its effect on weather patterns and on the very lives of millions of people around the world. It is a movement to raise questions and to listen to the prophets among us who are posing the difficult questions. It calls for affirmation of the reality of the situations that come to light, and intelligent recognition of their complexity and magnitude. It is the call to *be intelligent*, search for the values that move human activity, comprehend the difference between technologies that are life-enhancing and those that are not and know one's own gifts and limitations. *Being reasonable* is the facility to make judgments, to search for wisdom in the face of ambiguity and compromise. *Being responsible* is the call to individual and group initiatives—as simple as using less water for a shower, as threatening perhaps as addressing the anticaring structures of the places where we work and as broad-ranging as challenging the injustice of multinational corporations. In all, it is the human effort to restore at least a modicum of unity and harmony where chaos so often reigns. And as Lonergan adds, it is ultimately to be loving. Is this not the sum and substance of human care?

Alastair V. Campbell, in a 1984 study of the medical, nursing and social work professions, refers to professional care as *moderated love*. Reflecting on T.S. Eliot's *Ash Wednesday* (1934), Campbell suggests that

> professional care is one possible response to the fragmentation of our world, which expresses itself in illness and many other forms of social distress. The person who offers professional care seeks (perhaps unknowingly) to restore that lost unity, yet also inevitably shares in the fragmentation. Penitence, hope, realism and a search for lost harmony are all appropriate and necessary attitudes for people who aspire to care. Eliot's vision conveys them all (15).

The preceding reflections are grounded in an understanding of who we are as human persons, or perhaps better stated, who we are called and challenged to be. When our experience falls short of the ideals of human care, as often it does, we can take courage in its possibility as lived by caring mentors in the past and as demonstrated in the present by parents, family members, colleagues and patients, whom we encounter in professional life and practice. Perhaps at this time, at the beginning of the twenty-first century, when human life at all stages of development is in danger of being relegated to the status of property and commodity, when reification of human persons is the inevitable conclusion of experimentation without responsibility and when an individual's basic right to freedom for who she or he is as a unique, unrepeatable human person is bartered in the interest of science, we might find the basis for care and inspiration in the choice before Israel in Deuteronomy:

> I call heaven and earth today to witness against you: I have set before you life and death, the blessing and the curse. Choose life, then, that you and your descendants may live, by loving the Lord, your God, heeding his voice, and holding fast to him. For that will mean life for you, a long life for you to live on the land which the Lord swore he would give to your fathers Abraham, Isaac and Jacob (30: 19, 20).

2

CARING, THE HUMAN MODE OF BEING

We are acquainted daily with neighborly acts and acts of caring within our families, and among our colleagues and friends. We view on our television screens or in the news media the humanitarian efforts of groups in our own communities and all over the world. The world is not deficient in caring resources, be they human or financial. The response of persons to disasters affecting individuals, families and, on occasion, entire communities is generous and magnanimous; the gift of personal time and sacrifice is often heroic. In these instances, recovery is not only made possible because of the help of strangers, but it is fired by the physical, emotional and spiritual energy of people inspired by the experience of knowing they are being cared for. In the midst of devastation by whatever cause and of whatever magnitude, and in the experience of personal and family tragedy, we are touched in the depths of our souls by that sacred moment of knowing that we are in a world that is both communion and community. There are many examples of this truth.

In 1998, Hurricane Mitch completely devastated wide areas of Central America. The media coverage of this disaster led many to disbelief; some people to an apparent indifference, perhaps denial under camouflage; others to immediate action. Visitors representing the Canadian Catholic Organization for Development and Peace, the social justice arm of the Canadian Conference of Catholic Bishops (CCCB), visited the area and saw firsthand the personal, family and community effects of this hurricane. People lost family members and many relatives, were left without housing, and even their topsoil and means of livelihood. A call to the CCCB president generated an immediate response across Canada, raising eleven million dollars given directly to the people, and through their own community organization, was applied to rebuilding their homes and restoring their land. As the organizers of this project reported, "The way we responded changed our lives."

Nosotros, a videotape of recovery work primarily in Nicaragua, showed how men, women and children of the area, with generous financial support and energized by the concern of others, were able to restore their community and renew a way of life for what remained of their families and relatives. It is significant that, in the account of the experience, the people insisted they wanted to learn how to prevent similar tragedies and to acquire the necessary skills themselves to cope better with emergencies in the future. In the care people gave to and received from those providing help, the project, structured for their independence and the sustainability of their land, enabled them to put their lives together.

That same year, on 2 September 1998, the Swiss Air crash at Peggy's Cove, Nova Scotia, initiated an immediate and intensive response from the people of the small surrounding villages. The families, awakened at an early hour in the morning, did not stop to ask whether it was their responsibility to come to the rescue; response was instantaneous. Fishermen, who went out into the dark and misty fog with their small boats, were interested only in finding survivors and were devastated when they found no one. Residents' homes were opened to families and relatives who arrived in their village; hospitality was extended throughout the following year as family members, relatives and the people of Peggy's Cove tried to deal with an event that completely changed their lives. Reflecting on the response of fishermen, police, the military and ordinary people, Yvonne Vigneault, Congregation Leader of the Sisters of St. Martha of Antigonish, wrote to the editor of several Nova Scotia papers: "Thank you for showing to the world the human face of God, Maritime style." Peggy's Cove was but another of the many instances of communal connections, of being a family of human persons called to care. To go on with more examples would only be repetitive; the lived experience of communities everywhere continues this sacred story.

But even against the backdrop of these caring events, questions are sometimes raised as to the motivation of people involved—in whose interest? for what purpose? Are their actions genuinely altruistic or self-serving? On the one hand, we participate in and observe worldwide humanitarian efforts, the compassionate deeds of neighbors and friends and the heroic deeds of persons with special charisma and dedication. We think of Mahatma Gandhi, Albert Sweitzer, Mother Theresa, Jean Vanier, Tom Dooley, Jeanne Mance and a host of other persons who commit their life goals to making the world a better place in which to live. On the other hand, we have accounts of many people who give generously of their time and talents to their communities but do not necessarily see their activities as altruistic or other-centred. Does this admission come from genuine humility or self-effacement or from a sense that their actions are moved only by the need to promote personal gain and self-enhancing goals? I suspect such a clear distinction is not an easy one to make.

Robert Wuthnow (1991) speaks of an American paradox in a work based on a study, using in-depth interviews of one hundred persons, conducted in four regions of the United States. The sample was representative of men and women, younger and older people, with diversity in education and occupational backgrounds, religious affiliation and all, at the time of the study, involved in volunteer activities. The tension evident in the study between individualism and altruism in the American ethos raised concerns for Wuthnow: "In short, recent criticisms of American Society suggest that the delicate balance between individualism and altruism that has been part of our history may now be tipping in a direction that spells trouble for the well being of our nation" (20). The paradox is illuminated by statistics reported at the time of Wuthnow's study. Eighty million Americans were engaged in some kind of voluntary activity. The monetary value of unpaid volunteers in some areas of activity was estimated at $150 billion annually, and approximately 31 million people did volunteer work each year for their churches and synagogues. Wuthnow notes, however, that, while the level of volunteering and caring in American society suggests an image of wholesomeness, health, nurturing and goodness, "this Wonder Bread image of American society is only half the loaf, . . . There is another side to our character" (Ibid., 11). The other side is scripted by individualism and the accent on personal autonomy over altruism that, according to Wuthnow's study, shapes the values of American society.

Wuthnow focuses on what he sees as the problem in overemphasizing voluntary caring, of its being only a Band-Aid™ solution, which, at most, helps some people in need and brings to public consciousness the needs of others. But he argues that there is a great deal more to compassion than just helping the needy:

> Compassion is a value, a means of expression, a way of behaving, a perspective on society. We hope that it really meets needs, and everything possible should be done to facilitate it in meeting these needs. But whether it actually succeeds at that level or not, compassion still demonstrates our dependence on one another and gives us the hope we need to push ahead individually and as a society (308).

In a sense, Wuthnow's critique calls to mind the philosophy of a charismatic leader, Moses Coady, and the work of the Antigonish Movement that began in the difficult 1920s in eastern Nova Scotia. In responding to poverty and the complex social problems of people in the area, Coady espoused the value of community development through adult education and the cooperative movement, through which people became *masters of their own destiny* (1939).[1] Under his direction and working with his cousin, Father Jimmy Tompkins, the Extension Department of St. Francis Xavier University, Antigonish, Nova Scotia, was formally established in 1928. As did other movements, this one marked the response of individuals and communities of care to the needs of neighbors and, in particular, the poor and marginalized.

In a later chapter in this work, compassion is considered one of the ways in which human caring is expressed. Compassion is a way of entering into the experience of the other, of sharing in difficulty, pain and suffering, of being moved and changed by that experience.

One would hope that the response of people to Nicaragua, Peggy's

Cove, the Antigonish Movement and in many other projects throughout the United States, Canada and other countries is not simply volunteerism stripped of any semblance of altruism. On their own admission, people are changed by the experience. They claim to be better persons: their experience transformed their way of being with people and what they considered important in their lives, and there was a radical improvement in the social conditions that surrounded them. There was indeed personal growth and self-enhancement and, it seems proper to say, this happened through and because of extending themselves to others.

Wuthnow's study provides valuable insights, nonetheless, and prompts reflection on the motivating factors influencing vocational choice and everyday professional service. It has important implications for professional education. Why do we do what we do?

WHY IS REFLECTION ON HUMAN CARING IMPORTANT?

The stories surrounding Nicaragua, Peggy's Cove and the Antigonish Movement are but examples of what is going on among families and communities everywhere. These stories provide a lens through which we can see the goodness in people, the strength of communities and the reality of connectedness that binds a community of persons regardless of geographical location.

But there is also the dark side—another side to human experience. We live in an age where violence is commonplace. Atrocities are committed against individuals and communities everywhere. These are often the result of deliberate acts. Frequently, they are the indirect consequences of natural disasters and, sometimes, the result of a sequence of events brought about by unjust political and economic structures. The number of persons living on our streets is evidence of social dislocation involving family breakdown and abuse, unemployment, poverty and homelessness, and the breakdown of structures—however inadequate—which formerly provided a safety net. All of these experiences and events enter our living rooms through the press, radio and television almost as quickly as they happen. We have only to walk on the street and we encounter them personally. So frequent and repetitive is the occurrence that reports of violence and atrocities tend, on the one hand, to erode ordinary human sensitivities. On the other hand, they elicit responses by committed individuals and groups, initiating a growing swell of global, national and local outrage.

This age has special people but it also has less known caring, compassionate human beings—parents who nurture their children, families who care for their neighbors, politicians who commit their energies to furthering just political and economic policies, and many young people who enter the so-called "helping" professions because they care. While ours is a violent age, it is also an age with its own share of individuals and institutions dedicated to care.

Violence is not a new phenomenon in human history. But neither is the expression of human caring a new experience for humankind. History paints for us the ambiguity and seeming paradox of the human condition: the stark contrast between violent acts and compassionate deeds. The human race has survived because there has been a consistent number of caregivers and a continuity of caring. The human race has survived simply because of its humanity. "Man [woman] cares because it is his [her] nature to care. Man [woman] survives because he [she] cares and is cared for"(Gaylin 1976, 20).

The fundamental thesis of this work is that caring is the human mode of being. Caring is expressed in virtuous action and in habits acquired over time. It provides the energy that transforms doing things to and for people into service as ministry. Caring is not an exceptional human quality, nor the response of an exceptional few. Caring may be expressed with special grace and a unique quality by a special person or, indeed, may not be manifested or expressed at all. Nonetheless, caring is the most common, authentic criterion of humanness. Caring is humankind at home, not through dominating or controlling, but by being who we really are, being real, being true to self.

Milton Mayeroff (1971) deals with two basic themes in his work on caring: one, a generalized description of caring, and two, an account of how caring can give comprehensive meaning and order to one's life. He suggests that "the two concepts, 'caring' and being 'in place,' provide a fruitful way of thinking about the human condition; and what is more important, they may help us understand our own lives better"(2–3).

According to Mayeroff, caring qualifies our relationships with another and involves, most importantly, "letting the other grow" (2). Whether this other is a person, including oneself as other, an idea, an artwork or whatever, caring allows for growth, maturity and development. Caring is not possessive; it is not morbid dependence; nor is it dogmatically clinging to one's ideas. In the words of Mayeroff, we experience what we care for as having worth in its own right.

Mayeroff's discussion of devotion is also particularly relevant for persons in health and related services. According to his analysis, devotion is not an element that may or may not be present. Devotion is essential to caring: when devotion breaks down, caring breaks down:

> ... devotion does not simply measure the extent of my caring, but it is through devotion that caring for this other acquires substance and its own particular character; caring develops in the process of overcoming obstacles and difficulties. My devotion expresses my entire person rather than the intellectual or emotional part of me (8).

There are also obligations that derive from such devotion, obligations that we do not experience as forced on us. In the context of devotion, there is a convergence between what one wants to do and what one is supposed to do. Caring seems to place such value on the other, the task at hand, the challenge ahead, the immediate demand on time and energy, that the dividing line between wanting to and being obligated to tends to disappear and becomes irrelevant.

The human expression of caring may be shown through love or compassion, sorrow or joy, sadness or despair. It is humankind fired with zeal, concern or solicitude, or humanity bruised to the very core

29

of its being. Caring is the unique manifestation of a person's being-in-the-world.

Historically, some occupations and professions have been associated with caring or helping roles. We have referred to these as "helping" professions. Medicine, nursing and social work have been so designated. This manner of categorizing some occupations or professions as helping is problematic, however, implying that other occupations or professions by comparison are not helping. Such a distinction has tended to limit the scope and the understanding of caring to discrete functions, roles or tasks.

In the health care professions, care has sometimes been used as a characteristic to identify uniqueness or difference and to make distinctions on the grounds of such supposed uniqueness or difference. The designation of medicine as curing and nursing as caring is one example of this distinction and fortunately short-lived. Care must be a precondition for genuine cure (Nouwen 1974, 1979).

This work attempts to go beyond the pleasantries and the labels, the vocational slots and professional roles to an understanding of human caring as synonymous with being-in-the-world. It asserts that a person cares because he or she is a human being. The roles of auto mechanic, storekeeper, pastor, teacher, occupational therapist, social worker, nurse or physician are merely ways of living and acting through which persons in these roles live and express their human capacity to care. Knowledge, skills, experience and talent provide the props through which the actor lives out a uniquely human role on the particular stage of an occupation or a profession.

This work seeks to address the seeming paradox of the frequency of violence and absence of care with the claim that caring is essential to human development and survival. If caring is grounded in the human mode of being, the development of the capacity to care and be cared for is linked in unique ways to each stage of human formation.

In comparing animal and human gestation, Gaylin notes the complete helplessness of the human infant at birth. He asserts that "the most unique aspect of human development is the total helplessness of the human infant and the uncharacteristically long period of time in which it remains floundering in this helpless state" (1976, 31). Some animals face life at the moment of birth able to respond to the challenge of a new and sometimes hostile environment. Not so, the human infant. This dependency period, notes Gaylin, is "crucial to the development of the person who loves and is lovable, who has emotions and relationships, is capable of altruism and hope" (32). And he continues:

> If gestation is considered to extend beyond the year of birth, it is a peculiar kind of gestation, for it is the gestation of an aware fetus who, while helpless to act, is not helpless to perceive, and with that perception is learning lessons he [she] will never forget. Among these lessons, the most crucial one is the link between helplessness, care, and survival (33).

Caring is essential not only to the development of the human being but also to the development of the person's ability to care. The perceptions of the infant—the experience of love and warmth or lack of it—influence and shape the manner in which the person will relate to others as an adult. If the infant has learned to care through being cared for, the child has learned a crucial lesson in its journey toward full human development. An analysis of the relationship between helplessness, dependency, lovability and caring is provided by Gaylin (*see* 35–51).

Caring and caring relationships crucial to development are not one directional only. Human development is dependent not only on being cared for but also on being able to care. Human development and human fulfillment are achieved through the unfolding of the human capacity to care, through investment of the self in others, through commitment to something that matters. To have the capacity to care, however, does not automatically guarantee development, just as the capacity for intellectual acuity does not, in itself, create the intellectually astute person. The capacity to care needs to be nurtured, and such nurturing is dependent on its being called forth by others. Much human tragedy results when the human capacity to care is neither called forth nor expressed.

An interview by a CBC journalist of a man serving a life sentence for murder was aired on Canadian television some time ago. During the interview, the journalist asked about this person's possible involvement in another murder, where circumstances made him a suspect. In response to this question, the prisoner reacted with denial and spontaneous, violent rage, exclaiming: "When I was born no one cared; no one has ever cared, and I don't care." Rage, as a natural reaction of persons who have been abused or never been loved, is frequently the driving force of criminal acts. The reaction of this prisoner, who had been in and out of difficult home situations most of his childhood, is a telling manifestation of such a life-damaging experience.

> As light and visual stimulation are essential for the development of the capacity to see, so to be cared for is essential for the capacity to be caring. And to be cared for refers to all aspects of that word: to be taken care of, to be concerned about, to be worried over, to be supervised, to be attended to—to be loved (Gaylin 1976, 68).

Hope in the face of the human tragedy of failure to care lies in the capacity the human being has for change over time. Regardless of past experience, some people seem to possess infinite potential for modification and enjoy a wide range of possible responses. This reality is always a call to people in human services, but transformation of behavior and lifestyle can only be made real within relationships. As Gaylin has further stated:

> In order for each successive generation to fulfill its potential for becoming caring individuals, they must be treated in a caring way. We must be made to feel lovable in order to be loving. The degree to which we are nurtured and cared for will inevitably determine the degree to which we will be capable of nurturing and caring. . . . For this nurture supplies the stuff on which is built personhood, as well as person. Proper nurture will guarantee the development not just of an adult, but of a caring adult (50–51).

Caring as the human mode of being is also communicated in violent situations, in times of civil unrest and in the experience of war. Rollo May (1969) refers to a strange phenomenon about the Vietnam War communicated by photographs taken of that war: pictures of wounded caring for each other, of soldiers taking care of the injured, of a Marine with his arms around a wounded comrade, the wounded one crying out in pain and bewilderment. What comes back in the photo, notes May is "on this elemental level, care" (284). May describes the bewilderment equally communicated by the helpless child, face dirty with the smoke and soot from the smoke bomb, and the black American Marine looking down at the child. And reflecting on what may have been the thought of the Marine as he experienced this situation, May says, "I do not think [the Marine] ponders these things consciously: I think he only sees there another human being with a common base of humanity on which they pause for a moment in the swamps of Vietnam. His look is care" (285).

It is significant that, despite the abundance of material things possessed by so many people, material affluence is often experienced as hollowness, resulting in a prevailing hunger to be filled with more. There is a sense in which the mere possession of things, their appropriation to oneself destroys, at least temporarily, the very condition for the possibility of caring. In his analysis of this phenomenon, Rollo May reveals its roots in trends that are the antithesis of caring (1953, 41–69). These trends include the drive to competition, a loss of self and personal worth (being swallowed up in the herd), a loss of a language to communicate deeply personal feelings to each other and a loss of the sense of the tragic. All of these, in some way, reflect the person's inability to care—to care for oneself or to reach out to others. All of these inhibit the full development of individuals and communities.

This book involves research into the meaning of human caring in a culture where caring is more often known by its absence rather than by its presence in human affairs. When we experience violence, mistrust and human exploitation as the order of the day, we are moved to reflect on a question raised by many, the philosopher, as well as the person on the street:

> If indeed love and not hate or icy separation or indifference is the center of the universe, why is love so seldom observed in our world? Why is it that the law of the jungle, of power and strength and tooth and claw appears so often to be more central to our history and our human race than the practice of love? (Kelsey 1981, 38)

The Pitfalls of Research on Caring

Much of the violence we experience touches the lives of individuals and families with whom we are personally acquainted. To be academic about such an experience is almost to trivialize it. The reality of violence is so proximate and personal, and academia can be so detached and uncontaminated.

Another difficulty experienced in research on caring, and a reason for evading the discipline involved, comes from the exercise of the research itself. As we pursue a study of caring, we cannot help but note the discrepancy between the ideal—the inspiring thoughts and reflections—and the quality of our own relationships with self, with others and with God. The fear we may feel of being hypocritical or phony is a discomforting experience, and often it tends to become exaggerated. In my personal experience, this was a great stumbling block at a time when the urge to abandon the task of writing almost prevailed over the need to continue. This tension is experienced frequently by nurses and others in practice settings. They are persons who want to care, are professionally prepared to care, but are limited in their ability to do so because of conditions of the workplace.

While writing the first edition of this book, I had the privilege of spending a few hours with Henri Nouwen. In the course of our conversation, I spoke about the tension between caring relationships in everyday life and writing and lecturing about it. How do people bridge the gap between the ideals and concepts of caring and the realities of everyday experience?

Nouwen's response was clear and spoke to the importance of the caregiver caring for self. To succumb to the temptation to abandon a commitment because we begin to feel the reality of our limitations can be, in itself, a failure to care. This abandonment represents a failure to care for self through a compassionate acceptance of personal limitations. It is to bypass a moment of truth, to refuse a precious gift. Failure is not in itself weakness; failure occurs as a result of the refusal to grow through weakness. Is it not the case that the greatest growth periods in our lives are those marked by tensions that disrupt our comfortable patterns of living and relationships? As

Kelsey states, "The ultimate betrayal of life may well be the failure to love when one has the opportunity to do so" (1981, 25). This often comes as the call to love oneself.

In all of the preceding, it seems important to underscore the fact that, as wounded human beings, we do not become caring persons by reading scholarly theses; we become caring persons through hard work and intentional commitment, by engaging in the challenge of the virtuous life. I remember the words of a very wise high school teacher who would always respond to the panic of students before examinations by saying, "Work as if it depended on you; trust as if it depended on God." Nouwen's observation about compassion is relevant. We do not get a PhD in compassion. Rather it is a divine gift and the work of God's pure grace (Nouwen 1980; *see also* Nouwen et al. 1983).

Opportunities to care are not usually dramatic events. They most often come disguised in the simple, unobtrusive encounters of daily life—a smile, a helping hand, a word of encouragement and an expression of sympathy or, sometimes, in caring enough to reprimand. Arguments in support of research about human caring emerge from society's need for reflection on fundamental human values. They lie in the need to heighten awareness and raise human consciousness about the root causes of the value crisis in contemporary society. The person in a world that values technique and quick fixes is preoccupied with the question, What can I do? There is little time or place for, much less contemplation of, the question, Who am I? or Who should I become?

THE TWENTIETH CENTURY PARADOX: ENCOUNTER WITH THE DEMONIC

How can one claim that human caring is rooted in the very essence of one's humanity in face of the violence of the twentieth century, considered to be the worst in human history? How can a claim be made that caring is the human mode of being when a historical tragedy, the Holocaust, occurred during the lifetime of many of us, was carried out with demonic intensity and horror, wiping out millions of Jewish people because of who they were and others because of position or protests they held. It is said that the fact of the Holocaust itself marked the end of modernity. It negated any belief or hope in the cult of rationalism so strongly ushered in by the enlightenment. Unbridled reason had failed humanity.

Reading *Man's Search for Meaning* (Frankl 1959), for at least the third time, only increases within me a sense of shame and disbelief in the utter depravity of which we as human beings are capable. But Frankl's work does something else for most readers. As an account of dehumanization beyond imagining, it is also a powerful revelation of the high point of human possibility. As a profoundly inspiring and illuminating autobiographical account of the strength and triumph of the human spirit of the writer, it raises hope and belief in human goodness. It speaks to the potential human persons have at the core of their being for love, truth and wisdom.

Viktor Frankl, referring to the image of his wife separated from him on entrance to the concentration camp and, at that time, presumed to have gone to the gas chamber, reflects:

> A thought transfixed me: for the first time in my life I saw the truth as it is set into song by so many poets, proclaimed as the final wisdom by so many thinkers. The truth—that love is the ultimate and the highest goal to which man can aspire. Then I grasped the meaning of the greatest secret that human poetry and human thought and belief have to impart: The salvation of man is through love and in love. I understood how a man who has nothing left in this world still may know bliss, be it only for a brief moment, in the contemplation of his beloved. In a position of utter desolation, when a man cannot express himself in positive action, when his only achievement may consist in enduring his sufferings in the right way—an honorable way—in such a position man can, through loving contemplation of the image he carries of his beloved, achieve fulfillment. For the first time in my life I was able to understand the meaning of the words, "The angels are lost in perpetual contemplation of an infinite glory" (1959, 58–59).

Before going with a group to Russia a few years ago, and interested in Aleksandr Solzhenitsyn, I attempted to read *The Gulag Archipelago* (1997). Aleksandr Solzhenitsyn, who was awarded the Nobel Peace Prize for literature in 1970, was expelled from the Soviet Union in 1974 and lived in the United States until he returned to his homeland in 1994. Arrested in 1945 for making derogatory comments about Stalin, he spent eight years in labor camps. The Gulag, the abbreviation for *chief administration of corrective labor camps*, was the system that housed political prisoners and criminals of the Soviet system from the 1920s to the mid-1950s, where according to Solzhenitsyn, some forty to fifty million people served long sentences. I deliberately noted previously that I *attempted* to read *The Gulag Archipelago* because the horror that it described made it impossible for me to continue with the details.

Despite the dehumanization of Solzhenitsyn's experience in the Gulag and the harassment he endured on many counts, he continued to pursue the truth of his life and a commitment to reconciliation with the authorities of his own country. While in the United States, on 8 June 1978, Solzhenitsyn gave the commencement address at Harvard University. Expressing his gratitude for his stay in America and the hospitality he received there, he was rather blunt in his assessment of what he thought Western capitalism had to offer his country:

> But should I be asked, instead, whether I would propose the West, such as it is today, as a model to my country, I would frankly have to answer negatively. No, I could not recommend your society as an ideal for the transformation of ours. Through deep suffering, people in our country have now achieved a spiritual development of such intensity that the Western system in its present state of spiritual exhaustion does not look attractive. Even those characteristics of your life which I have just enumerated are extremely saddening (34–35).

On his return to Russia in 1994, he was greeted with euphoria as he stepped off the train at intervals during his travel to Moscow. During one such stop, while in conversation with an individual in the group, another, pointing to the person talking with Solzhenitsyn, protested, "He was one of the KGB." Solzhenitsyn replied by reminding him that it was now time for reconciliation.

In Western culture, Viktor Frankl and Aleksandr Solzenhitsyn stand tall as luminaries, both as victims of cultures that had lost their souls and, within those cultures, as models of triumph of the human spirit, as signs of hope for the possibility of preserving human dignity and goodness. Fortunately, the witness of such persons serves as a reminder that the call and prospects for shaping a better world are open to all people of goodwill and determination. The lives of recognized saints used to do this in the past. Perhaps we need to reclaim this heritage and also look more intentionally for the unsung heroes in our midst. The following Roman myth is food for reflection.

> Once when "Care" was crossing a river, she saw some clay; she thoughtfully took up a piece and began to shape it. While she was meditating on what she had made, Jupiter came by. "Care" asked him to give it spirit, and this he gladly granted. But when she wanted her name to be bestowed upon it, he forbade this, and demanded that it be given his name instead. While "Care" and Jupiter were disputing, Earth arose and desired that her own name be conferred on the creature, since she had furnished it with part of her body. They asked Saturn to be their arbiter, and he made the following decision, which seemed a just one: "Since you, Jupiter, have given its spirit, you shall receive that spirit at its death; and since you, Earth, have given its body, you shall receive its body. But since "Care" first shaped this creature, she shall possess it as long as it lives. And because there is now a dispute among you as to its name, let it be called "homo," for it is made out of humus (earth) (Heidegger 1962, 242).

A Conceptualization

The following conceptualization of human caring—always tentative—is a slightly adapted version of that in the original monograph (Roach 1984). It is an overview of the essential components of this work. While highlighting nursing, it is not intended to exclude other health care professions and occupations.

1. Caring is the human mode of being.

2. An individual cares not because of his or her particular role but because he or she is a human being.

3. Caring is essential to human development. One becomes fulfilled as a human person as one's capacity to care is called forth, nurtured and appropriately expressed.

4. The capacity to care, while it may be repressed or suppressed, is almost indestructible.

5. Caring is not simply or exclusively an emotional or feeling response. Caring is a total way of being, of relating, of acting; a quality of investment and engagement in the other—person, idea, project, thing, self as "other"—in which one expresses the self fully and through which one touches most intimately and authentically what it means to be human.

6. Caring is responsivity—response to value as the important-in-itself.

7. Caring is professionalized in nursing and in other helping professions through affirmation of caring as the human mode of being, and through development of the capacity to care through the acquisition of skills—cognitive, affective, technical, administrative—required for the fulfillment of prescribed roles.

8. Caring is the virtuous life, expressed explicitly through such attributes as compassion, competence, confidence, conscience, commitment and comportment.

9. Caring is not unique TO nursing in the sense that it distinguishes nursing from other professions or occupations. Rather caring is unique IN nursing in the sense that, among other characteristics descriptive of nursing, caring is unique. It alone embodies certain qualities; it exists as the sole example of specific characteristics. Caring is the locus of all attributes used to describe nursing.

10. Preparation for service professions, which seek to professionalize the capacity to care, presupposes a curriculum based on a holistic, integral humanism and an environment for teaching and practice where caring models are visible.

11. Individual women and men select nursing as a career because they desire to help people—to care for people. A commitment to nursing and to other service professions with the personal and professional fulfillment it brings presupposes the ability and freedom to care.

12. Nursing and other caring professions evolved within Judeo-

Christian and other faith traditions, embodied a virtuous way of life and were inspired by faith in an all-loving, all-compassionate God.

13. Within contemporary society, where Judeo-Christian values and the values of other faith traditions are in sharp tension with a prevailing materialistic and naturalistic humanism, the nursing profession is discovering and/or recovering its traditional raison d'être and its inherent values. Central to this revisiting is the emergence and the centrality of human care.

14. Professions came into existence as society experienced the need for more formally organized human services to respond to the need to care and be cared for. Health professions continue to evolve as professions as they respond in their own unique ways to this need of society and of their own members.

Endnotes

1. Other works on the Antigonish Movement include: A.F. Laidlaw, *The Campus and the Community*; J. Lotz and M. Welton, *Father Jimmy: Life and Times of Jimmy Tompkins*; A. Alexander, *The Antigonish Movement: Moses Coady and Adult Education Today*.

3

REFLECTIONS ON CARING ATTRIBUTES

In preparation for the first edition of this work (1987), clarification of the concept of human caring came from many sources—the experience of caregivers in education and practice, the ordering of ideas in curriculum development and observations about what caregivers do when they are caring. The question, What is a nurse doing when he or she is caring? elicited a wide range of specific responses. In order to arrange these responses in a manageable order, the SIX Cs were structured. The study, however, raised a large number of other questions that needed to be addressed.

THE CARING UNIVERSE

The following categories were chosen to allow for diversity in focus and provide logical areas of inquiry for this work. The use of such categories may by instructive in understanding human caring as it is in itself, may facilitate development of models for inquiry into caring actions and may be useful for the articulation of education and learning in the caring sciences generally. Such categories have been helpful for the writer in understanding the originality, as well as the complementarity, of the growing body of literature on caring from various perspectives of research in both education and practice.

1. *Ontological.* Ontology is an inquiry into the being of something

and into its range of possibilities, and asks the questions: What is the being of caring? What is caring in itself?

2. *Anthropological.* Anthropology poses such questions as, Is caring rooted in and claimed as a value in the cultural identity of people? How is human caring expressed among different peoples and cultures?

3. *Ontical.* Onticology refers to the study of some entity in its actual relation with other entities. Examples of ontic statements include normative statements about how one wishes to live, statements of obligation, factual statements and questions (*see* Schmitt 1969). In this category, I include the functional and ethical aspects of caring. What is a person doing when he or she is caring? What obligations are entailed in caring?

4. *Epistemological.* Epistemology is concerned with ways of knowing. Questions in this category include, What are the different ways in which caring may be known, observed and expressed?

6. *Pedagogical.* The pedagogical category is concerned with teaching and learning and the strategies used to facilitate specific learning needs and goals. How is caring learned and taught?

The purpose of identifying a caring universe as a way of posing questions relevant to areas of study is simply to clarify the approach and focus of this particular work. A comprehensive treatment of each is not intended. While some reflections may relate to all categories—the nature of caring as such; what it means to be a caring person; caring functions and behaviors; the knowing, teaching and learning of caring—, these categories are not dealt with systematically. The main purpose of the work is to engage the reader in a process of reflection and inquiry about caring as the *human mode of being*, about human caring as expressed in virtuous acts and to assist in naming one's identity as a professional person intentionally committed to care.

While caring ontology is the overriding theme throughout this work, this chapter focuses on the ontical category. As noted previously, ontic statements include normative statements about how one wishes to live; statements of obligation; expressions of one's "Weltanschauung;" how one incurs moral guilt; factual statements, questions in science and factual statements of everyday personal and professional life. Functional and ethical manifestations of caring are included in this category.

THE SIX Cs

The SIX Cs of Compassion, Competence, Confidence, Conscience, Commitment and Comportment evolved over time in response to the question, What is a nurse doing when she or he is caring? At this level, specific manifestations of caring, as represented by such behaviors as taking the time to be with, checking factual information, identifying and using relevant knowledge, performing technical procedures, showing respect, maintaining trusting relationships, keeping a commitment and comportment in dress and language were generalized into the SIX Cs. These are referred to as attributes of caring and, while not mutually exclusive, serve as a helpful basis for the identification of specific caring behaviors.

Before beginning this second revised edition, a session was arranged with members of the nursing practice committee of St. Martha's Regional Hospital, Antigonish, Nova Scotia. In consultation with the nurse manager of intensive care, palliative care and progressive care units, a case study was prepared and presented to a group of seven, ranging in experience from fifteen to thirty years. While this case study was not identified exclusively with one particular patient, patients, family and staff on these units commonly experienced the elements highlighted in the study.

The purpose of meeting with members of the nursing practice committee was to obtain feedback on how they see their nursing role as individuals, as members of a team, and to determine what they considered to be the call it represented to nursing in general. To allow for a spontaneous response to the case study, without the influence of bias from my work, the nurses were not given material on the SIX Cs prior to the meeting. To my knowledge, no one had used my work on caring, at least not recently.

Each nurse was asked to read the case study and, without discussing it with anyone else, reflect on what this situation called forth in her personally and from nursing in general. After observations were shared, each nurse was asked to discuss the case with a person next to her. A group response was then solicited and both personal and group responses were recorded. After a short break, a brief overview of the SIX Cs from the original work was presented, and the group was then provided with a form on which they would record responses.

THE CASE STUDY

Mrs. D., a fifty-two-year-old woman, is a patient in PCU following admission from emergency three days ago. She experienced pain in the upper left quadrant for four days prior to admission and has had poor appetite and weight loss for several months. She is experiencing lethargy and nausea and, while the pain is under control, she complains of much abdominal discomfort and has little desire for food. Her husband and three adult children are regular visitors, revealing a closely knit family. A medical consultation with the family has just concluded, and the surgeon has related to them the seriousness of Mrs. D.'s condition, noting she has a malignant, inoperable tumor of the pancreas. He assured them everything will be done to keep her as independent and comfortable for as long as possible. Given the progression of her condition, he advised consultation with palliative care and proposed plans for home care, with pain and symptom control. The nurse attending the conference noted the anxiety of the family and the desperate emotional state of the husband. There is obvious disagreement among family members about disclosing the diagnosis to their mother who has a family history of cancer. However, the oldest daughter, a social worker, insists the mother should be given all the facts about her condition, noting her strength and ability to deal with her illness. The other family members disagree, resisting contact with palliative care and pushing the husband to a more protective role, including nondisclosure. A fourth family member has been away from home for several years and has not maintained contact. The father is attempting to trace his whereabouts. He stated this son was "mother's favorite," and often, recently, Mrs. D. has talked about him.

The process with members of the nursing practice committee was carried out in a limited period of time, approximately one hour and thirty minutes. The responses were spontaneous and speak for themselves. While the final group response was undoubtedly influenced by an overview of the SIX Cs, it was shaped primarily by their initial reaction to the case study. In a letter of appreciation, participants were given written feedback and a copy of the chapter of the book on the SIX Cs. I inquired about the accuracy of my summary and invited their comments on the experience. But I did not make a return visit.

Responses revealed much consistency, highlighting the following issues: family involvement and patient-family interaction, truthfulness, the need for information, patient rights, symptom control and the need for all involved to have an opportunity to participate and communicate feelings. The response of the group as a whole was characterized by a relational quality, with strong emphasis on health-team and patient-family involvement. The following is a verbatim summary of specific responses.

Compassion.
- Attempt to experience what patient is experiencing.
- Patient and family are experiencing the hardest thing possible—loss of someone they love.
- Need of family to adjust—the patient may already know.
- Recognize loss of patient and family; respond appropriately.
- Recognize patient-family needs to express fears, expectations.
- Recognize family-patient needs.

- Feel for feelings of family members and patient.
- Allow expression of "desperate emotional state;" must be a very difficult thing to hear about.
- They may not have much time; help them come to reality of situation.

Competence.
- Must know what the condition is about, how treated, what is available to the patient.
- Know how to orchestrate each program and guide patient and family through it.
- Importance of experience, understand this illness to be able to treat symptoms, physical, emotional, etc.
- Be able to assess, plan, implement and evaluate a plan of care to meet needs of patient-family.
- Be aware of upcoming deterioration of condition; support both patient and family.
- Understand what patient-family may need physically, emotionally, etc., over next while.
- RNs-team have knowledge and skills, communication in guiding patient-family.
- Knowledge and experience relative to this diagnosis.

Confidence.
- I must instill in the patient and family a feeling of confidence.
- They have to trust me to give them good information and advice.
- We must show that we have the tools to make Mrs. D. comfortable.
- Trusting in my ability as a nurse, based on sound knowledge and experience.
- Expressing this confidence enables a trusting relationship between nurse-patient-family.
- Instill in patient the awareness that you are there for her and for her family.

- Comfortable with self (personal qualities, skills).
- Comfortable and open with family and patient.
- Enable freedom, aware of risk of taking over for patient-family.
- Inform, encourage support of all aspects of care.
- Provide holistic care.
- Sensitive to ethics. Truthfulness is a big part of this. If truth is brought forward it gives a trusting relationship with patient and family.
- Confidence in trying to bring family together.

Conscience.
- Trust self and do what I think is right in this situation.
- Always advocate for the patient.
- Conscience tells me the patient needs to know about her condition; let her decide how to handle it.
- Sensitive, informed sense of right-wrong important to realize that Mrs. D. has a right to know her condition.
- Intuitive knowing what to do or how to respond appropriately.
- Helping patient and family to sort out how they are feeling and what their needs are.
- Patient must be allowed to put her needs first.
- Morals—fine-tuned with knowledge and skills.
- Understand patient's rights.
- Important to let patient know so she can make decisions re her condition and care.
- Patient needs to know at appropriate time.
- Know patient's rights; ensure they are not violated.
- Re ethical decisions to be made; refer to health care team.
- Keep informed of ethics-standards.
- Know that everyone deals with grave situations differently; deal with everyone as an individual.

Commitment.
- Sticking with patients through crisis.
- Realize ongoing relationships with family; will be with us until patient dies.
- As nurses we can help Mrs. D. and family come to terms with her illness.
- Staying for the duration and being available when needed.
- Letting them know you are committed to them.
- Do not give in to the easy way out.
- Be there to allow all to express their fears and be an avenue to unite all in a central focus.
- Convergence between what you want to do and what you ought to do.
- Being able to help family come to consensus so that you-they can be open to patient.
- Commitment first for the comfort of the patient and, second, for the whole family, not excluding the patient.

Comportment.
- Look and sound like the professional I profess to be.
- Be true to myself and to the patient.
- Important to portray ourselves in a certain way.
- Show patient and family we respect them.
- Show patient and family who you are by your dress, manner and actions.
- Always show respect for patient first, disease second.
- Present yourself as someone who demands respect.
- Always have a way about you that gives family and patient the ability to respect you and, therefore, be comfortable with your knowledge and skills.
- Showing the patient and family that I care how they come together for comfort of patient.

In writing the account of my session with members of the nursing practice committee of St. Martha's Regional Hospital, I became conscious of the fact there was no mention of spiritual care, at least, not specifically articulated. I did not build into the process a question relative to spiritual care per se, and I suggest the apparent absence of their attention to this important facet of care was conditioned by the nature of the process itself. This hospital has a strong commitment to its mission and identity as a Christian institution within the Roman Catholic tradition and has a plan for the integration of mission at all levels of its activity. With a vibrant and active Department of Religious and Spiritual Care, with staff and volunteers available to persons of all denominations and faith traditions, there is no doubt the spiritual needs of this patient and family would have been a priority.

Suggestions for Reader Participation

The following reflections are offered to the reader as background for further consideration, noting how caring manifests itself in everyday health service, in practice, education, administration and research. If one is interested in doing so, it might be helpful to revisit the case study. The following questions are a suggested guide only.

1. What is going on?
   - Identify the issues, problems and dilemmas (if any).
2. Who is involved?
3. What values are explicit, implicit in the narration?
4. What knowledge, affect, skills are required to care for this patient and family?
5. What knowledge, affect, skills do I bring to this situation?
6. How is caring as virtue—as my way of being with this patient and significant others—in this particular situation called forth?
7. What implicit, explicit boundaries does this case study raise for me? For nursing? For health care in general?
8. What is transpiring within myself?
9. What do I wish to be, to become as a person, in my caring ministry?

A Further Elaboration of the Six Cs

Compassion

Compassion may be defined as a way of living born out of an awareness of one's relationship to all living creatures. It engenders a response of participation in the experience of another, a sensitivity to the pain and brokenness of the other and a quality of presence that allows one to share with and make room for the other.

In his writings, Henri Nouwen offers key insights on compassion. Of particular significance are reflections he shared with me in the spring of 1980 and published in a work (Nouwen et al. 1983). The word "compassion" is derived from the Latin words pati and cum, which together mean to suffer with and involve us in going

> where it hurts, to enter into the places of pain, to share in brokenness, fear, confusion, and anguish. Compassion challenges us to cry out with those in misery, to mourn with those who are lonely, to weep with those in tears. Compassion requires us to be weak with the weak, vulnerable with the vulnerable, and powerless with the powerless. Compassion means full immersion in the condition of being human (4).

The resistance this kind of commitment evokes, notes Nouwen, shows that compassion is a much less obvious human virtue than we might be led to believe. It is in discussing this point that Nouwen parts company with some of the contemporary philosophical discussions of caring. He identifies compassion as the radical quality of the Christian life, the call to "be compassionate as your Father is compassionate" (Ibid.). But like contemporary philosophical treatises on caring, Nouwen also asserts that it is ultimately through compassion that our humanity grows into fullness.

While working on one of his books, Nouwen and a number of his colleagues visited U.S. Senator Hubert Humphrey to discuss his views on compassion in public life. Humphrey, considered to be one of the most compassionate men in the political life of his time, was more than a little surprised by the purpose of Nouwen's delegation. When he learned of their mission, Humphrey moved from his large desk to a small coffee table in his office. Suddenly, he walked back to his desk, picked up a long pencil with a small eraser at its end and said,

> Gentlemen, look at this pencil. Just as the eraser is only a small part of this pencil and is used only when you make a mistake, so compassion is only called upon when things get out of hand. The main part of life is competition: only the eraser is compassion. It is sad to say, [Humphrey continued], but in politics compassion is just part of competition (1980, 5–6).

The being compassionate as your Father is compassionate is translated into a call to imitate God's particular way of being with us, God-with-us. According to Nolan (1978), the New Testament account of the miracles of Jesus is evidence of his identification with the suffering, the poor and the outcast, and he notes "[A]nyone who thinks Jesus' motive for performing miracles of healing was a desire to prove something, to prove that he was the Messiah or Son of God, has thoroughly misunderstood him. His one and only motive for healing people was compassion" (35–36).

For the Christian, compassion is participation in the compassion of the Godself. It is this participation that provides an antidote for the kind of competitiveness that reduces compassion to the soft eraser at the end of a long pencil, something used only when we make mistakes. Seen within the context of a radical call to the Christian life, compassion becomes our second nature, our natural way of being in the world.

Compassion is a relationship, lived in solidarity with others, sharing their joys, sorrows, pain and accomplishments. Compassion involves a simple, unpretentious presence to each other, a gift that we seem to have lost even as we have developed sophisticated techniques in our efforts to acquire it. Thus, we cannot go far with commercialized compassion or calculated kindness. For, as Nouwen insists, we do not acquire compassion by advanced skills and techniques. According to his analysis, we receive compassion as a totally gratuitous gift.

As Nouwen (1980) further observes, one of the most tragic events of our time is that we know more than ever before about the sufferings and tragedies of the world, yet we are less able than ever before to respond to them. Perhaps in reflecting on this disturbing reality, we might ponder his insistence that

> [c]ompassion is not a skill that we can master by arduous training, years of study, or careful supervision. We cannot get a Master's degree or a Ph.D. in compassion. Compassion is a divine gift and not a result of systematic study or effort. In a time of so many programs designed to help us become more sensitive, perceptive, and receptive, we need to be reminded continuously that hard work is the fruit of God's pure grace. Therefore, if there is a discipline of compassion, we must understand it as a human response that makes visible a divine gift that has already been given. In the Christian life, discipline is the human effort to unveil what has been covered, to bring to the foreground what had remained hidden, and to put on the lampstand what had been kept under a basket. . . . It is the revelation of God's divine spirit in us (132).

Matthew Fox (1979) considers compassion to be the "world's greatest energy source," and a way of life. He examines compassion from the perspectives of human sexuality, psychology, creativity, science, economics and politics, and from its central place in the healing of the global village. He asserts that "compassion has been exiled in the West. Part of the flight from compassion has been an ignorance of it that at times borders on forgetfulness, at times on repression, and at times on a conscious effort to distort it, control it and keep it down" (1).

Introducing his analysis with a reflection on what compassion is not, Fox observes that compassion is not pity but celebration; not sentiment but making justice and doing works of mercy; not private, egocentric or narcissistic but public; not mere human personalism but cosmic in its scope and divine in its energies; not about ascetic detachments or abstract contemplation but passionate and caring; not anti-intellectual but seeks to know and to understand the interconnections of all things. Compassion, says Fox, is not religion but a way of life, that is, a spirituality; not a moral commandment but a flow and overflow of the fullest human and divine energies; not altruism but self-love and other love at one.

The following summary by Fox is helpful:

> Compassion may be a passionate way of living born of an awareness of the interconnectedness of all creatures by reason of their common Creator. To be compassionate is to incorporate one's own fullest energies with cosmic ones into the twin tasks of 1) relieving the pain of fellow creatures by way of justice-making, and 2) celebrating the existence, time and space that all creatures share as a gift from the only One who is fully Compassion. Compassion is our kinship with the universe and the universe's Maker: it is the action we take because of that kinship (34).

In reflections on compassion, Gula accents care for self as well as care for others.

> Compassion is the virtue which enables us to value the other for himself or herself and not for some functional or utilitarian means to our end.
>
> The heart of compassion is living patiently with others while seeking their well-being. It begins with heeding our own self-care that nourishes our physical, emotional, spiritual, and moral health. Staying healthy frees us to accept ourselves so that we can be for others without projecting onto them our own needs, fears, and illusions. . . . The virtuous love of self includes neighbor love because we can only come to fulfillment as part of a community of love. Appropriate love of self frees us to meet the needs and to protect the freedom of the vulnerable (1996, 46).

That compassion is an attribute of caring hardly needs defending. In an age where the scientific and the technological are weighed heavily and often considered the norm for human progress, there is a need to emphasize the humanizing ingredient of compassion and "for the cold and impersonal world of science and technology to be infused by things of the spirit" (Hellegers 1975, 113).

James Conlon speaks about the spirituality of the earth, the compassion of the earth, about compassion as woven into the fabric of life. Compassion is about experiencing communion and the energy of interconnectedness, supporting the harmony and balance already woven into earth. "Our open invitation is to experience compassion, to fall in love with ourself, with each other, with Earth and the cosmos, to become vulnerable, open, connected" (1994, 54). In contemplating the embrace of the earth, attend to the following exercise suggested by Brian Swimme. On a clear night, lie on the ground and look up toward the stars. Close your eyes and imagine you are looking down on the stars, because actually you are. What is holding you to the earth? What is keeping you from falling? What does it mean to be held in the embrace of the earth?

COMPETENCE

For purposes of this discussion, I shall define competence as the state of having the knowledge, judgment, skills, energy, experience and motivation required to respond adequately to the demands of one's professional responsibilities.

Compassion, indispensable to the caring relationship, presupposes and operates from a competence appropriate to the demands of human care. While competence without compassion can be brutal and inhumane, compassion without competence may be no more than a meaningless, if not harmful, intrusion into the life of a person or persons needing help.

There was a time when some people, including individuals within the nursing profession, considered kindness and a strong physique as the major requirements for entrance into the occupation of nursing. If this opinion was ever justified, and I suggest it was not, there is no doubt that the demands of nursing today require more than kindness and a strong constitution. Practice in all service professions requires a high degree of cognitive, affective, technical and administrative skills, with specific competency requirements in each of these areas. Professional caring demands such competence.

One of the threats to caring competence in our day is the misconception and misuse of power. This threat spells the difference between competence as a manifestation of caring, and competence as manipulation—as an expression of human violence. The power that is human violence is symbolized by Fox's reference to the up-the-ladder syndrome. In his terms, this syndrome is manifested by an up-down, Sisyphian, competitive, restrictive, elitist survival of the fittest and hierarchical mentality toward living in a world where there can be only winners and losers. It is this kind of power that stifles our capacity to care. In the words of Fox, "When one is climbing a ladder one's hands are occupied with one's own precarious survival and cannot be extended to assist others without putting one's climb and even one's life—if one is high enough upon the ladder—into jeopardy" (1979, 49).

It is a power wielded by compulsive people, driven to power, driven to prestige, driven to possessions. It is a kind of power that reflects a restrictive dualistic way of thinking, seeing life's situations exclusively in terms of black-white, either-or, fixed-mutable, science-religion, male-female, conservative-liberal, and so forth. Fox reminds us that this dualism is the ultimate lie that undermines all possibility of compassion in the world. And this threat is experienced at a time when we need, perhaps more than ever before, a greater consciousness of the interconnectedness of all things, of a way of seeking both-and, and of a way of living characterized by a letting be, a letting go and a letting dialectic happen (85–103).

But caring does indeed demand competence. The ability to care, and to care appropriately and adequately, requires that we have the freedom to learn and the opportunity to practice in our respective professions in a manner compatible with the dignity and needs of those we serve. We should not have to do this, however, at the expense of someone else. We should not have to do it within a power struggle, which suffocates the very source of caring energy, a power struggle that is exemplified by the drive to be at the top of the pyramid. Are there power struggles in your workplace? What effect do they have on team spirit, on the freedom of caregivers to care?

Being-in-the-world, being-for-others is authentic when it calls the other to freedom; it is inauthentic when characterized by dominance and depersonalization. The mature use of power does not preclude respect for self, nor does it imply the relinquishment of legitimate personal autonomy. It implies an understanding of competence tempered by a compassion that is "the ultimate and most meaningful embodiment of emotional maturity," and through which a person "achieves the highest peak and deepest reach in his or her search for self-fulfillment" (Jersild 1957, 201).

Confidence

The term confidence is defined as the quality that fosters trusting relationships. It seems impossible to think of caring without, at the same time, thinking about the importance of a trusting relationship. It is equally impossible to imagine achieving the goals of service without, at the same time, assuming that the service will be rendered within an environment and under conditions of mutual trust and respect. Much is being done in professional disciplines to foster trusting relationships. But, while confidence might be considered as a given, its absence in the world of everyday affairs creates the need to examine the quality of its presence in the service fields.

In a work by Sissela Bok, the author speaks about the decline in public confidence in the United States. Bok notes:

> The loss of confidence reached far beyond government leadership. From 1966–1976, the proportion of the public answering yes to whether they had a great deal of confidence in people in charge of running major institutions dropped from 73 percent to 42 percent for medicine; for major companies from 55 percent to 16 percent; for law firms from 24 percent (1973) to 12 percent; and for advertising agencies from 21 percent to 7 percent (1979, xviii).

There does not seem to be strong evidence that this situation has changed much for the better during the time since the last edition of this work was published. Frequent litigation infers a rapidly increasing climate of mistrust within the professions, as well as in society as a whole, and a brief search of material on-line reveals the extent of concern about trust and confidence in public institutions. (Global concerns are raised in Pharr and Putnam [2000].)

Duplicity in public life appears under many guises. Duplicity in health care, according to Bok, is similarly camouflaged, in some cases, with deliberate deception in care, and experimentation and research treated casually or with indifference. In relating to this phenomenon, Bok notes the lack of stress on veracity in medical codes, for example, and examines the arguments used to rationalize and justify lying to clients. Codes of ethics for research, particularly those receiving public funding, do provide a safety net, however, and guidelines are there to increase awareness and sensitivity to the violence of human trespass.

The 23 March 2001 edition of the *Toronto Star*, carried the following headline, "Medical Students Pressured to Be Unethical: Survey." According to this report by Helen Branswell, Canadian Press, a survey of medical students at the University of Toronto Medical School "found nearly half had been put in situations where they were pressured to act unethically by their teachers." The situations, as reported, included doing examinations on comatose or anesthetized patients without their consent; without consent, doing procedures for teaching purposes that did not have to be done; and having patients make unnecessary return visits to clinics for teaching purposes only. The associate dean, responsible for the undergraduate medical training program, responded to the coverage by saying the British medical journal which published the report had done the profession a service. Noting the University of Toronto was no different and certainly no worse than any other school, the focus was welcomed as a means of drawing attention to the issues, and as a reminder that patients could no longer be taken for granted in teaching hospitals. The university has taken steps to strengthen ethics education.

Fidelity to canons of loyalty, to the ethical standards in teaching situations in teaching hospitals, can be on very fragile ground. The attitude that patients admitted to teaching hospitals *know they will be used for teaching and could go elsewhere* is not uncommonly expressed. The tension between teaching and the learning needs of students in all health disciplines and the service-care requirements of patients and families has been ever present. The issue is not *no more patient-centred learning* but attentiveness and fidelity to the virtue of caring in all situations, acknowledging the patient-family as partners in the educational enterprise, not objects to be used. This obviously presumes respect and always consent.

It is not within the parameters of this work to do a comprehensive study of health care codes of ethics. But reference will be made in a subsequent chapter to challenges to canons of professional ethics as guarantor of, or even as a reliable norm for, ethical practice (Pellegrino et al. 1991; Brockett 1997). A brief statement from the Canadian Nurses Association *Code of Ethics for Registered Nurses* is of interest here.

> The nurse-client relationship presupposes a certain measure of trust on the part of the client. Care and trust complement one another in professional nursing relationships. Both hinge on the values identified in the code. By upholding these values in practice, nurses earn and maintain the trust of those in their care (1997, 5).

The use of deception is one issue that still remains both a threat and a topic of controversy. Regardless of the weight of the arguments used for distorting the truth, or the complexity of the problems with which the caring profession has to deal, I still make the claim that deliberate deception—even the co-called "white lie"—not only shatters the confidence of the client but also damages the integrity of the professional as well. Deception destroys confidence; deliberate deception is the antithesis of caring.

Caring confidence fosters trust without dependency, communicates truth without violence and creates a relationship of respect without paternalism or without engendering a response born out of fear or powerlessness. Confidence, then, is a critical attribute of professional caring.

Conscience

Conscience, understood as the morally sensitive self attuned to values, is integral to personhood (*see* Maguire 1978). Conscience reflects the sacredness of the person, points to the sacred core of the personality and to the centre of personal integrity. Conscience is the voice where the claim of the one is asserted over the power and the persuasion of the many. Conscience is the medium through which moral obligation is personalized.

This is not to claim that conscience is simply a matter of personal opinion and, as such, supersedes the collective moral perceptions of the group. Individual conscience must be sensitive and informed. Individual and collective consciences are not adversaries; it is not a question of one or the other. Moral judgment requires the wisdom of both.

Conscience is related to the whole structure of one's being—to care. Authentic existence by definition is acting in accord with self and conscious awareness; inauthentic existence is not acting in accord with such awareness. Care, as primordial, is the foundation of moral consciousness (*see* Heidegger 1962).

Moral norms, standards, principles and values, grounded in religious faith, shape our actions by enlightening reason and enable us to reflect on and articulate the values by which we live. A further examination of conscience as an ingredient of our reflection and formative in decision making may help us understand the movements of that process.

Most persons experience conscience, "My conscience tells me." "My conscience bothers me." But, as universal as the experience of conscience may be, individual variation and misperceptions are commonplace. The *Canadian Oxford Dictionary* uses the Latin derivative conscientia (knowledge) and conscire (to know or be privy to) (s.v. "conscience"). When the word is broken down into its two derivatives—cum (together) and scientia, scira (to know)—it includes not only knowledge and awareness but *together* as well. This latter interpretation offers an understanding of conscience as connoting a relationship—persons as social and communal: "Conscience is the person's moral faculty, the inner core and sanctuary where one knows oneself in confrontation with God and with fellowmen [women]. We can confront ourselves reflexively only to the extent that we genuinely encounter the Other and the others" (Haring 1978, 224).

Psychology helps to clarify the understanding of conscience, particularly in the distinction made between it and the superego. In the Freudian school, the superego is interpreted as the policeman of the personal life, regulating behavior strongly influenced by guilt. Gula (1989) likens the superego to the attic of a house where all the "shoulds" and "have-to's" are stored. Regulating behavior from the fingerpointing authorities of the past, in overdependency on being loved and approved, the individual is moved only by external rules, demands and guilt fixations. Reductionist views eliminate conscience as a factor in shaping behavior, emphasizing instead conscience dependent on training according to social norms or domination by the superego. "The moral conscience, on the other hand, acts in love responding to the call to commit ourselves to value" (126).

O'Connell (1976) provides three helpful distinctions: Conscience: general sense of value, awareness of personal responsibility, capacity for self-direction, human responsibility for good direction. Despite cultural differences in interpretation, "all human persons share a sense of the goodness and badness of their deeds" (89). Conscience: exercise of moral reasoning; identification and perception of values; involves reflection, discussion and analysis. At this stage, all that shapes our lives and ways of thinking influence decision making. Even when we bring to this process the sincerity of honest judgment, however, we can be wrong. We need the assistance and insights of others, the wisdom of the past and objective voices from the church and society. To make responsible moral-ethical decisions, our conscience needs to be educated. Conscience: concrete judgment pertaining to immediate action.

Gula (1989) parallels the preceding distinction describing conscience as 1) capacity—one's fundamental ability to discern good and evil, 2) process—as the discovering of what makes for being a good person, what particular action is right or wrong, the process of being formed and informed, and 3) judgment—following inquiry and leading to judgment. And Gula remarks, this will be as reliable as the homework we do to inform it.

The word conscience is defined as a state of moral awareness; a compass directing one's behavior according to the moral fitness of things. As an expression of caring, conscience entails responsivity, expressing itself as a response to something that matters, a response to a value as the important-in-itself. It involves the spiritual power of affectivity.

The writer D.C. Maguire considers affective reaction to value to be the "foundational moral experience" (1978, 84). Conscience is "the morally conscious self in his [her] acute state of moral awareness" (371). Affective response is not equated with emotivism or mere feeling states. It is an intentional response, deliberate, meaningful and rational. In locating moral consciousness in love and caring, Maguire relates the following incident from anthropologist Loren Eisley:

> Anthropologist Loren Eisley, starting from the existence of the one-armed skeletal remains of a Neanderthal man, offers an imaginative reflection that is relevant:
>
> Forty thousand years ago in the bleak uplands of south-western Asia, a man, a Neanderthal man, once labeled by the Darwinian proponents of struggle as a ferocious ancestral beast—a man whose face might cause you some slight uneasiness if he sat beside you—a man of this sort existed with a fearful body handicap in that ice-age world. He had lost an arm. But still he lived and was cared for. Somebody, some group of human things, in a hard, violent and stony world, loved this maimed creature enough to cherish him.
>
> Somewhere there in the period of harsh beginnings, there appeared, in Eisley's words, loving, caring, and cherishing. Concern was born and with it morality.... What it was was the light of a distinctively human consciousness, animated by the unique energy that we have come to call love. This ability to appreciate and respond to the value of personal life in all its forms is the foundation of moral consciousness (85–86).

Conscience is the caring person attuned to the moral nature of things. Conscience is not simply a thing added on at some point in one's experience. Conscience grows out of experience, out of a process of valuing self and others. Conscience is the "call of care and manifests itself as care" (Heidegger 1962, 319).

The particular state of moral awareness that constitutes the self at any given time is fallible; its claim on right and wrong is not absolute. In an experiential sense, no one realizes this fact more than the person who struggles to understand the moral implications of human relationships and the moral status of the actions of human beings on one another. Professional caring demands that our moral awareness be fine-tuned by the discipline of knowledge and moral inquiry. Professional caring is reflected in a mature conscience and is understood to subsume the moral-ethical imperatives and norms of professional life.

Commitment

For the purpose of this discussion, commitment is defined as a complex affective response characterized by a convergence between one's desires and one's obligations, and by a deliberate choice to act in accordance with them.

A work on educational objectives—affective domain (Krathwohl et al. 1964)—provides helpful insights on the internalization of values. Of particular significance is its placement of commitment on a continuum where internalization of a particular value is recognized as well established. Commitment presupposes or goes beyond other behavioral responses such as willingness to receive, willingness to respond, an acceptance of a value and a preference for a value. In this work, commitment is considered to be evident when choice is so firm that what one commits oneself to do is synonymous with what one prefers to do. Commitment becomes part of one's identity as a professional, caring person.

In Mayeroff's philosophical analysis, caring is considered to subsume the quality of devotion. According to this analysis, in devotion, as noted previously, there is convergence between what I want to do and what I am supposed to do. Devotion (commitment) is essential to caring: if devotion (commitment) breaks down, caring breaks down. Commitment is a quality of investment of self in a task, a person, a choice or a career, and therefore a quality that is so internalized as a value that what I am obligated to do is not regarded as a burden. But rather it is a call that draws me to a conscious, willing and positive course of action.

The everyday experiences of persons in health care are shaped by many forces and conditions; some are obvious, others are not. While it is individuals who make commitments, the latter are always influenced by social factors. The health care person brings to work on a given day concerns of family and of personal relationships. And the ability to care itself may be nurtured or hampered by the work environment and constraints of the system. Perhaps Mayeroff's reminder of the reality of human limitation—there are a limited number of persons, projects and things to which we can commit ourselves at any given time—helps to take these realities into account. In speaking with groups of nurses, emphasizing this point has often been sufficient to diffuse a false guilt. To realize one's limits in the ability to care and to be compassionate toward self can create the energy caregivers need to care even more.

A work by Farley (1986) provides a comprehensive study of personal commitments—beginning, keeping and changing. While Farley's work is beyond the scope of this book, her ideas around commitment, love, promise-keeping and, in the context of faith, of covenant are most helpful. In her discussion of forms of commitment, she identifies what she calls a " 'prime case' a central form of commitment—one from which all other forms derive some meaning. Commitment to persons, when it is explicit and expressed offers such a 'prime case' " (15). An ethic of care, caring as relational responsibility, presupposes a commitment to persons.

A further distinction Farley makes about the nature of commitments is also enlightening. There are commitments to truth, to values such as the institution and family life; to justice, beauty and peace; to plans of action; to be a good parent; and to live in accordance with the Gospel. But the common meaning that keeps these values from becoming empty, abstract ideals is willingness to do something. And then there are commitments that may be total or partial. Total commitments involve the whole person, raise identity issues about who one really is and desires to be and constitute fundamental life options. These may be marriage and family or a choice of a vowed life in a religious order. Partial commitments may include a professional choice, a job or position. In consideration of such distinctions, perhaps the greatest challenge of persons committed to care is to determine priorities and acknowledge limitations in all of them. No attempt is made here to even suggest solutions to a call that is, in reality, a life task.

At any given moment, we experience different levels of commitment and varying degrees of difficulty in being faithful to the choices we believe we ought to make. Some responses do not require reflection and are so internalized they are almost automatic. A good parent, for example, does not deliberate at 3:00 a.m. whether he or she should respond to the needs of the sick child. Response is an unquestioned and implicit convergence between what the parent wants to do and what he or she ought to do. It is an expression and a manifestation of who she or he is as a person, as a parent. At other times, whether the matter is trivial or seriously complex, a decision requires deliberate reflection and choice may be more difficult. As with the other Cs, commitment is always the challenge that caring demands.

COMPORTMENT

The idea of comportment as an attribute of caring emerged from a discussion with a competent, committed clinical nurse specialist. This person expressed concern and uneasiness over what she observed in the dress and language of nurses while caring for patients. The problems involved sloppy dress and inappropriate language, and the concern and uneasiness came from the unfitness of both to the caring image of a professional caregiver. Comportment, meaning bearing, demeanor or to be in agreement or harmony with, served as an appropriate attribute to subsume these kinds of concerns. It must be noted, however, that the interpretation and use of the word comportment in this context is more restricted than its meaning of *overall commitment*, as sometimes used.

Dress and language are symbols of communication and can be in harmony or disharmony with a caring presence. When we visit a special person, our mode of dress and choice of language are usually in accord with the regard, esteem and respect with which the person is held. Without necessarily reflecting on the matter, we usually dress and use language consistent with our attitude toward the person or the occasion. We dress appropriately and observe certain socially accepted protocols when we accept an invitation to a garden party at Buckingham Palace, the White House or the residence of the governor general of Canada.

In the past few decades, as a reaction or, perhaps, even a protest against conformity to former rigid standards of dress, there has been a radical change to a more practical choice of uniforms appropriate to different situations. Speaking of nursing, Kaiser refers to studies indicating that by the mid-1970s, "the traditional nurse's uniform had become increasingly ineffective as professional clothing, for several reasons" (1985, 372). The reasons included a general decline in the prestige of uniforms and an emphasis on "power" dressing among professionals in the larger culture. Many nonprofessional workers' dress resembled that of nurses—the latter thus losing their sense of identity—and greater numbers of men entering the nursing profession. Increasing numbers of nurses were found in more diverse clinical roles and management positions.

But we also experience the shadow side of change, sometimes with an "everything goes" mentality, and less demonstration of what even social grace might require as "professional attire." In some situations, dress codes seem more difficult to establish and even more difficult to adhere to. I suggest we need to reflect on whether such a trend is consistent with our stated beliefs about the dignity of persons, including ourselves as professional caregivers. How does observance of social etiquette in the situations noted previously transfer into regard for the patient, family, colleagues and others? Given the nature of current practice, I suggest this question deserves honest reflection at all levels of the health care professions. We might begin by asking, Are dress and language of caregivers consistent with the belief that the patient-client is of incalculable worth, and that the caregiver him-/herself is a person of intrinsic worth and dignity?

Caring is reflected in bearing, demeanor, dress and language. An inquiry into the symbolism of dress and language and their relationship to professional caring could be an interesting area for research. According to Kaiser's study, appearance continues to be an important sign of "legitimacy" and identity for health care workers. Perhaps the central question is, What does clothing mean? What signs and symbols does dress communicate? And considering there are other signs that communicate something about who we are, Kaiser continues,

> [Y]et clothing is one of the most eloquent and powerful products we use; it is an expressive medium, or concrete way revealing particular ideas in the mind that cannot be otherwise articulated. The object and

sign are linked in a way that is highly visual, connected intimately with the person (owner), and conducive to every social dimension of daily life (219).

Summary

Reflections on the attributes of professional caring presented in this chapter are intended to cast light on the range of possibilities of human caring from the ontical perspective. They are presented as goals that we are always striving to achieve. Given the woundedness experienced by all persons who desire to live the virtuous life, we are not always where we want to be, and we fall short of the expectations we have of ourselves. Such occasions provide a test for the quality of compassion we have toward ourselves.

The ontic category addresses such questions as, How does one wish to live? What obligations are entailed in particular choices? What constitutes caring in the everyday life of a professional person? What is a person doing when he or she is caring? No attempt is made here, however, to deal with these questions in such a manner as to arrive at precise, specific answers. The exercise of responding to a case study was a simple way of drawing out the caring capacity already present and operative in the nurses who composed a nursing practice committee of a regional hospital. It was not designed as a controlled research study.

The SIX Cs are used as a broad framework, suggesting categories of human behavior within which professional caring is to be understood. In compassionate and competent acts; in relationships qualified by confidence; through informed, sensitive conscience; through commitment and fidelity; and in a manner of dress and language in harmony with held beliefs about the dignity of persons, specific manifestations of caring are actualized. Behavior expressed by the SIX Cs says a great deal about personal identity. Most importantly, such a way of virtuous acting encompasses much of what a professional person wants to be.

4

CARING AND PROFESSIONAL ETHICS

A nursing program in the 1940s at St. Joseph's Hospital School of Nursing, Glace Bay, Nova Scotia, had as a required text, *Ethics and the Art of Conduct for Nurses*, by Edward F. Garesché (1929). One theme in this text, noblesse oblige, made an indelible impression on me; and it has surfaced repeatedly as a value in presentations to groups about ethics or related topics. Perhaps, noblesse oblige hovers over my reflections about nursing because it conveyed something of the beliefs about nursing at that time and most likely the particular motivation behind my personal choice.

The text by Garesché covered central concerns of ethics in health care in the 1940s, including the nature of human acts, the importance of conscience formation, professional secrecy (confidentiality) and general attributes expected of one preparing to become a nurse. The specific content covered by this course, however, eludes my memory, perhaps because the phrase noblesse oblige subsumes it all. This phrase made the claim there was something about nursing in itself which was noble, and if one chose to pursue a nursing career, such a choice involved assuming a particular identity. As this work attempts to reflect and communicate, the nursing identity is acquired through the professionalization of the human capacity to care, an identity shaped by the virtue of caring and expressed through a way-of-being in relationship.

While, at present, we do not use the language of noblesse oblige, I suggest related desires and values move persons to choose nursing today. The motivation of entry-level students continues to be fired by a desire to care and, while societal values such as self-interest, individualism and a materialistic culture suggest otherwise, the reasons of the majority of persons entering nursing are expressed as, "I want to care for others." Women and men choose a health care profession because they want to care for people. This observation has been born out in my experience as a nurse educator and, in later years, as both patient and colleague in relationship with medical and nursing practitioners whose primary desire is to care as professional persons. This desire is at the heart of their professional lives, whether practitioner, teacher, researcher or administrator, despite the trappings of role and the confinement and constraints of the system.

Health care is a moral enterprise. It is a moral enterprise because it brings persons into unique relationships. Whenever we are in a relationship with another person, we establish bonds and these bonds, grounded in trust, entail duties and responsibilities—an ethic of relational responsibility. When we studied ethics in the 1940s, the content, examined in the context of health care in the twenty-first century, was relatively simple. Nonetheless, I propose the values subsumed under noblesse oblige still hold, if not take on greater significance.

What is the basis for believing the quality of relationships of caregivers emanates from an understanding of a profession characterized by nobility, health care actions as human acts of a noble character and human caring itself a virtue? This chapter is an attempt to underscore the ethical-moral call for the professions as we embrace the challenges in the new millennium. Hopefully, reflecting on who we are and why we are in health service will continue to inspire us to ride above role fixations. Focusing on our identity as persons committed to virtuous caring activity can provide the energy needed to challenge barriers within the system including the identification of health care services with market values, political and financial gain. Attention given to ethics helps to shape and monitor a way of life that enhances health care as a service both to caregiver and to recipient. This chapter focuses on the background and context for ethical-moral reflection.

Introduction: Understanding the Language

Ethics (morality) is concerned with human behavior and relationships, with standards, moral rules and the values by which we live. Etymologically, the words *ethics* and *mores* are derived from the same root meaning. In practical usage, however, these words take on a different connotation. For example, ethics may refer more strictly to principles, standards and guides for action; morals to action itself. In this work, the terms ethical and moral will sometimes be used interchangeably; the primary context for ethical-moral reflection is relational.

The word ethics is derived from the Greek, ethikos; the word moral from the Latin, mos, mores, both literally translated to mean custom. The customs to which ethics and morals refer, however, are specific types of customs. Some customs are conventions, fads or fashions including table manners, modes of dress, forms of speech and expressions of social grace and courtesy. Customs embrace etiquette—conventional forms and usage—, matters of decorum suggesting dignity and the sense of what is becoming or is appropriate and propriety, implying established conventions of morals and good taste (Fagothey 1976).

Ethical and moral customs differ from conventions, fads, fashions or matters of protocol. They are considered not only customary but also right, reflecting neither a passing whim nor social convention but abiding personal and communal values. Ethical-moral customs are discovered, not invented, constitutive of the moral fabric of human communities within a civilized society.

But moral behavior is not guided exclusively by rules; our actions reflect who we are as persons. "Moral goodness is a quality of the person, constituted not by rule-keeping behaviour alone, but by cultivating certain virtues, attitudes, and outlooks" (Gula 1989, 7). Moral reflection and the responses we make to ethical-moral concerns and challenges call on the whole person and, while requiring knowledge and rational discernment, embrace the values and beliefs, the virtues and habits that shape us as human persons. In critiquing human response, one cannot separate person and action.

By nature, the human person is drawn to the good, but as personal and communal experience demonstrate, the good is not always easy to discern and frequently not chosen. We may take refuge in the words of Paul, "I cannot even understand my own actions. I do not do what I want to do but what I hate" (Rom. 8:15). Nonetheless, we are challenged as human persons to live a good life. How, then, do we arrive at an understanding of the good and the good life?

CARING, ETHICS AND THE MORAL LIFE

A study of ethics may be approached from different perspectives: 1) as a discipline of knowledge, 2) as relational responsibility and 3) as a process of discernment.

ETHICS: DISCIPLINE OF KNOWLEDGE

As a discipline of knowledge, ethics content is highly weighted in theories, principles, moral rules and standards. Accrued over centuries, ethics as a discipline has focused on the good, the good life and how to live it, and draws from traditions of philosophy, theology and religious studies. What was identified as the good and the good life varied from the free exercise of intelligence in the pursuit of truth, to stoicism, to a life of pleasure, to utility and to what is in keeping with human nature.

Contemporary ethical discussion is frequently focused on complex cases and on the more dramatic issues that make the news media. Questions usually concern what should be done, what makes for the best decision, under specific conditions at a particular time and place, all of which are important elements in decision making. The values that animate discussion around such issues vary, are sometimes controversial and raise conflicting claims. As an example, the principle of autonomy, interpreted as the right to self-determination, may be antithetical to other communal values involving persons in relationships of family and society. An individualistic position on human rights may consider assisted suicide a claim on the health service system. But the principle of beneficence, of do not kill, dictates otherwise.

Recent studies focus on virtue ethics and ethics of character, on the way of life of persons in relationships. This attention to virtue ethics raises an almost forgotten, if not denied, source of ethical reflection for consideration and, in the process, enlightens discernment. Virtue ethics, while not a new invention, is coming to the forefront in dialogue and current literature. (*See* MacIntyre 1981; Hauerwas 1981; Shelp 1985; Patrick 1996; Keenan 1998; Spohn 1999.) The publication edited by Shelp (1985) covers a wide range of positions, including an historical analysis, theories of virtue, and virtue and medicine, and concludes with a critique. It is not possible to cover the wide range of views in these resources. A few comments show its relevance for this work.

The Greek word for virtue, arete, is interpreted as an excellence that denotes the power of something to fulfill its function. As a combination of excellence and power, virtue would seem to be that which enables us to fulfill our function as human beings. In the introduction to this work, caring is seen as the virtue at the heart of who we are as human persons, and as the core value that inspires, directs and sustains nursing's identity and the identity of all persons who choose professions of care. It models for us a desirable good. Hauerwas notes "An ethic of virtue centers on the claim that an agent's being is prior to doing" (1981, 113). He further states:

> What is significant about us morally is not what we do or do not do, but how we do what we do. A person of virtue is often said to be a person of style or class in that he or she may well do what others do but in a distinctive manner. Nevertheless, virtue is not the same as "style"; we associate virtue with a more profound formation of the self (Ibid.).

We are not always comfortable with reflections on virtue ethics as the following experience shows. In the late 1970s, I had the privilege and challenge of directing a code of ethics project for the Canadian

Nurses Association. It is interesting how many persons questioned how I, as a Roman Catholic and member of a religious order, could be *objective* or at least not enforce my personal values on the process. There was a sense that the personal and professional were completely separate and had to be kept so, and what was done on off-duty time should have no bearing on practice. It would seem that it was imperative to separate the private person from the person who happened to be a professional. This did not mean, however, that Canadian nurses across the country did not share the common values that shaped their professional lives. The unease over the relationship between private and professional persona, however, became a major concern as far as the content of the code was concerned. This tension continues as an even greater challenge in contemporary society.

The final outcome of the code of ethics project, based on study and consultation with ethicists, moral philosophers, moral theologians and members of the profession across Canada, was a proposed code of ethics (Roach 1981), accepted initially by the CNA's board of directors. The core value of the code was *caring*; its underlying principles were *sanctity of human life* and *respect for persons*. Its final disposition is a matter of history. The main point here is that, as individuals and as profession, we had certain perceptions and expectations about what should be included in a code of ethics. An articulation of a virtuous, personal life and shaping how we practiced as professional people was not at that time highlighted as one of these expectations.

Virtue ethics does not bypass a discussion of ethical theory or systems, but its foundational questions are focused on person and character such as, Who am I? What person ought I to become? How do I get there? (Keenan 1998). It focuses on the standards and values by which we live and on the place of virtue in our lives. "Rather than examining actions and asking whether we should perform them or not, virtue ethicists say that persons ought to set ends for the type of people they wish to become and pursue them" (86). In the words of Pellegrino (1985), "the contemporary appraisal is not an abnegation of rights or duty-based ethics, but a recognition that rights and duties notwithstanding, their moral effectiveness still turns on the disposition and character traits of our fellow men and women" (238). Most importantly, attentiveness to virtue ethics may well prevent us from overlooking the distortion of our moral sense or of not adequately articulating such by an ethic devoid of virtue (Hauerwas 1985).

In a critique of Western philosophy from the Enlightenment on, MacIntyre (1981) makes the observation that we possess "fragments of a conceptual scheme, parts which now lack those contexts from which their significance derived. We possess indeed simulacra of morality, we continue to use many of the key expressions. But we have—very largely, if not entirely—lost our comprehension, both theoretical and practical, of morality" (2).

There are differences of opinion as to where virtue ethics fits and the place it ought to have in ethics in both dialogue and practice. My sense is that the fire, which provides the energy for the values we hold, the principles and moral rules by which we live, the needed foundation for any theoretical position whether deontological, teleological, rights ethic or all combined is generated in and by virtue. I suggest an ethics of virtue fills the void in an approach to ethics as a rational process only and sheds new light on the imperative for nursing, that is, noblesse oblige. And ethics of virtue is consistent with the choice of nursing in the first place, with the motivation of those who imagine themselves as persons of care.

ETHICS: RELATIONAL RESPONSIBILITY

A focus on ethics as relational responsibility does not contravene the importance of principles, values or moral norms. Neither does it bypass the process of discernment. It is distinguished primarily by the contextual approach it uses, with participation of all persons involved.

In his reflections on what he describes as the Catholic natural law tradition, Gula (1989) speaks of natural law as an approach to discovering moral value through reflection on the totality of human reality and experience, "reason reflecting on human experience discovering moral value" (241). It takes into account the call of persons, their duties and obligations in the context of life's purpose and goals. We might ask, What moral values surface in one's experience, for example, as a nurse, physician, technologist or parent? And how do these values shape the call to care? What impact does living a virtuous life of caring for self and others have on one's sense of self, on everyday relationships in marriage and on human flourishing? (*See* Cahill 1996.)

H. Richard Niebuhr (1978), in a critique of deontological and teleological theories, for so long the core of ethical theory, suggests an alternative way of perceiving and living the moral life. He proposes the symbol of person as *answerer*, engaged in dialogue and acting in response to an action of others. This symbol of the person as answerer is at the heart of Niebuhr's ethics of responsibility. The teleologist asks the question, What is my goal, ideal or telos? prior to determining what ought to be done. The deontologist asks, What is the law and what is the first law of my life? Responsibility proceeds in every moment of decision and choice to inquire: "What is going on?" (60). An ethic of responsibility involves response, response in accordance with interpretation of the question to which an answer is being given, and accountability that, according to Niebuhr, includes anticipation of answers to our answers and social solidarity. He further adds:

> The idea or pattern of responsibility, then, may summarily and abstractly be defined as the idea of an agent's action as response to an action upon him in accordance with his interpretation of the latter action and with his expectation of response to his response; and all of this is a continuing community of agents (65).

Niebuhr provides a dynamic context for ethical critique and discernment for all persons in health care, embracing a broad range of questions from the daily activities of the caregiver, to organization and strategies of management, to dominant operational thrusts within the health system itself.

Bernard Haring (1978) speaks of responsibility as the leitmotif, the leading theme and norm that permeates and elucidates all norms, ideals and goals. He proposes a responsibility essentially marked by liberty, fidelity and creativity set in contradiction to an exclusive focus on duty. Responsibility proceeds from a vision of wholeness in which it perceives the value and meaning of human life. Within a biblical perspective, Haring notes the centrality of God's call and covenant, and the human person's response in fidelity and gratitude for God's liberating action and fidelity to covenant. The accent is on relationship. The starting questions in Haring's concept of responsibility are not, first of all, What ought I to do? but What ought I to be? and What is the makeup of a responsible, creative person? A further emphasis on this concept is found in an understanding of the covenant relationship (Gula 1996).

Covenant or contract. We may arrive at a better sense of covenant by comparing it with contract relationships with which we are familiar. In our everyday lives, in positions, civil arrangements, in buying and selling, we are accustomed to making and signing agreements or contracts. Contracts protect the parties involved, attempt to ensure honesty and are intended to prevent one party from taking advantage of the other. The contract spells out in advance what I must do to receive something else. Gula makes an important distinction:

> When we act according to a covenant we act beyond the minimum. A covenantal relationship accepts the unexpected; it makes room for the gratuitous, not just the gratuities. Partners in a covenant are willing to go the extra mile to make things work out. Covenantal thinking wants to know what is the most we can do in grateful response to what we have received. This makes sense when we realize that the original context of the covenant is a gracious God who loves freely and without end (1996, 15).

In a 1997 work, Roach notes a paradigm case in a study of the experience of ethical issues by nurses in critical care nursing (Fenton-Comack 1987). The narrative is about a nurse who goes the extra mile in caring for a dying man of unknown origin and address, admitted from the streets to a large inner city hospital. The nurse stays with this man after her scheduled hours as she was the only person who could be with him when he died. This nurse had already fulfilled her contract with the hospital; she also, perhaps, without even reflecting on or using the word covenant or without any conscious religious motivation, transcended her contract by entering into a relationship of love for another human being.

> He has nobody to be with him when he dies. It made me feel very rewarded. I felt in some ways pleased that I could be with him. He did not have to be alone. He opened his eyes occasionally and he knew someone was there and I held his hand (195).

Speaking of the relational nature of human persons—generally, specifically and uniquely—Keenan (1998) enumerates the key demands made by a life grounded in virtue:

> [A]s a relational being in general, we are called to justice and to treat all people fairly; as a relational being specifically, we are called to fidelity and to sustain the specific relationships that we enjoy; as a relational being uniquely, we are called to self-care that no one else can provide (92–93).

In specific terms, caring is living in the context of relational responsibilities—responsibilities to God, to self and to the other. Whether practitioners, educators, researchers or administrators, activities involve us in human relationships that imply responsibility to ourselves, to patients, families, peers and colleagues. To the extent that these relationships are inspired and shaped by human care, to that extent are they consistent with the ethical norms of relational responsibility.

In his book, *The Patient as Person*, Paul Ramsey speaks of these norms as canons of loyalty, using the biblical notion of fidelity to covenant as the model. Ramsey considers the moral requirements of medical ethics as only a particular case of the moral requirements governing the relationships between human beings. He states: "We are born within covenants of life with life. By nature, choice, or need we live with our fellow men [women] in roles and relations. Therefore we must ask, what is the meaning of faithfulness of one human being to another in every one of these relations? This is the ethical question" (1970, xii).

Ramsey notes the aim is "simply to explore the meaning of care, to find the actions and abstentions that come from adherence to covenant, to ask the meaning of sanctity of life, to articulate the requirements of steadfast faithfulness to a fellow man" (xiii).

ETHICS: PROCESS OF DISCERNMENT

As process, ethics shifts back and forth from a deductive approach, using principles, moral norms and standards as a way of discerning the right-appropriate action, to an inductive, contextual approach, focusing on *what is going on* in the lives, morals and values of persons as both inquirers and participants. In other words, process as contextual, while calling on moral rules and ethical principles, considers the moral life as more than the application of rules, standards and principles but as life lived by persons in community. The noblesse oblige of nursing or other "helping" professions is one expression of the sacredness of this contextual reality of both those who serve and of persons and communities served.

The decisions we make and the values that shape our lives do not come from some innate body of knowledge or from values that we procure in the same manner as we buy our clothes or food in the marketplace. Responsible moral-ethical decisions are not simply preferences or matters of opinion. They are formed within a process of discernment, grounded in knowledge pertinent to the matter in question, and the values that shape our lives and are constitutive of virtuous living. There is integration of content, situation and context.

Ethical decision making in health care presupposes astute clinical expertise. But the complexity of the issues we face calls for a breadth of knowledge in all areas of concern and, most importantly, the wisdom of all engaged in the process. It involves ongoing discernment as the focus for seeking the good—the good in this situation, the individual good, the common good—and addressing the unique and specific demands of human care. No one is expert in everything; all persons living out of an awareness of mutual dependency have the capacity to meet the moral-ethical challenges of our time with honesty, integrity and, above all, humility. A mature conscience, at least one always on the way to maturity, is an essential ingredient in the process. (Conscience was addressed as one of the SIX Cs in chapter 3.)

Use of models for ethical-moral discernment. A formal model for ethical discernment is not always necessary, especially when ethical issues and problems are straightforward and frequently attended to. Ethical discernment becomes a habit that serves one well in everyday health care practice. This is not to say that habitual moral responses are automatic, nonreflective ways of acting, but rather the fruit of virtuous living. Both desire and the practice of human care become a way of life. We realize this fact acutely when we experience uncaring moments in our relationships with others.

There are occasions, however, when the problems experienced are more complex. Their complexity is accentuated by the realities of a society of moral-ethical pluralism, experiencing a disaffection with principles and rules, while at the same time revealing a need for standards by which to live and practice. The process of discernment is also hampered by a reductionist ideology that detaches ethics from any association with faith or religious experience. Within the working environment itself, where decision making often takes place while on the run, appropriate response to the moral issues and problems encountered daily is further compromised. So a guide, if not imperative, serves a purpose. If nothing else, it clarifies use of language.

In the multifaceted, tangled web of moral-ethical challenges, confusion is lessened and the course of action clearer, if descriptive labels of events or situations are accurate. If we have to act on our feet, and frequently this is the case, it helps to have a clear perception of what we are dealing with. In others words, What is going on? What are the real issues? A distinction between an ethical issue, an ethical problem and an ethical dilemma provides some clarity in identifying the elements of these issues.

In both oral and written communication, the word dilemma is often used as an umbrella term for ethical challenges regardless of the factors involved in the situation. This general use of the word creates ambiguity in understanding the problem and colors the direction or procedure thought to be necessary in moving toward a responsible course of action. Wright (1987) provides a helpful clarification. In a situation assessment procedure, Wright notes, "An issue identifies an area of concern, regardless of whether there is a problem present"

(51). (*See also* 44–63.) It differs from an ethical problem. Confidentiality, always an ethical issue, does not become an ethical problem until information given in confidence is at risk of disclosure. For example, an airline pilot in a visit to his doctor discovers he has a serious heart problem and asks the doctor not to disclose this information to his employer. The ethical problem arises because nondisclosure of information normally kept confidential puts at risk a third party, in this case, the crew and public. The challenge for the doctor, as well as the pilot, is to determine how the public is to be protected and who discloses what information and to whom. In distinguishing ethical problem from ethical dilemma, Wright defines an ethical dilemma as a situation "in which no matter what a person does, the result will be something which is not desirable" (52). While ethical problems may be complex and difficult to resolve, they are not dilemmas by definition. The use of the principle of double effect is helpful for attending to such issues (CHAC 2000, 13).

Along with clarification in the use of language and assessment of relevant questions, effective ethical decision making, while not bound by any particular model, follows a systematic procedure. Given the realities of time and urgency, however, it is important to have some ordered way of moving through difficult and complex situations. Within the context of human caring as virtue, this always involves discernment of the good, for others and for self. (Available models can be found in *Reason and Conduct* [Aiken 1962]; *Human Values in Health Care* [Wright 1987] and *Health Ethics Guide* [CHAC 2000]).

Reflections on caring as a guide for discernment. Revisiting the case study in chapter 3, against the background of these reflections on caring and professional ethics, gives rise to the following questions.

1. What affect does the caregiver bring to this situation?
2. In what manner does noblesse oblige, an awareness of the sacred space in which health care is lived and practiced, move and influence the caregiver, including members of the family and significant others?

3. How does a covenantal relationship differ from the contractual arrangements of all caregivers?
4. How does the caregiver blend personal and professional life in objective ethical discernment?
5. What is going on? Who is the central focus of this case?
6. Who are the participants in this community of care?
7. As moral community, what are the duties and responsibilities of all involved?
8. How do the virtue of caring and virtuous acts shape and direct the care of this person, as member of family, as patient in hospital?
9. What are the key areas of concern, that is, ethical issues?
10. What ethical problems are surfacing?
11. Are there dilemmas for caregivers, for the patient, for family members?
12. What moral rules need consideration, for example, truth-telling, honesty, confidentiality, do not harm, promise-keeping?
13. What are the relevant ethical principles, for example, respect for persons, sanctity of life, autonomy, justice?
14. How do faith, religious values, the mission of the organization or program influence the course of discernment?
15. As members within a moral community of care, who do we desire to be, to become?

The suggested questions are offered as an aid to identifying the actual and not so visible factors in the life of this patient and her family and, hopefully, help to shape dialogue and response. It is a process always open to discovery and, in faith perspective, experiencing the presence of the God of compassion in the relationships of this community.

Summary

In itself, the case study in chapter 3 and the response to it model the SIX Cs. In entering into the experience of patient and family, as well as that of colleagues, the capacity to care is called forth in compassionate acts. The caregiver applies knowledge and clinical expertise within a climate of relational responsibility, bonded in covenant.

5

PROFESSIONS, PROFESSIONALISM AND TRUST

Since the time when professions were limited to ministry, law and medicine, many other occupational bodies have become involved in self-examination and identity issues relative to their professional status. The formal criteria for inclusion were: 1) possession of a body of knowledge, 2) commitment to service, 3) self-regulation through codes of ethics and 4) enjoyment of rewards that symbolized accomplishments sought as ends in themselves (Barber 1963; Freidson 1986, 1988; Kultgen 1988; Pellegrino et al. 1991). The focus of this chapter is on professionalism as the foundation for reflection and discernment on matters of trust. It is not an historical overview of the evolution of professions, even though professions continue to be the object of redefinition (*see* Malin 2000; MacDonald 1995; Abbott 1988; Freidson 1986).

Within the reflections of this study on caring ontology, perhaps the debate over whether a particular occupation is a profession is not a prior issue. Occupational groups or so-called semiprofessionals, through the acquisition of knowledge and skill, and commitment to service, define themselves by who they are and how they pursue their goals. The call for all is to *professionalism*—to be caring persons maintaining a sense of integrity, authenticity and self-identity in the face of economic pressures, the constraints of the marketplace and the controls of a system shaped by bureaucratic values and managerial structures.

In the introduction to his work, Malin notes "[T]he sociological literature on professions has largely treated the values associated with professionalism—altruism, personal detachment, public service, etc.—as part of the rhetoric by which professionalizing groups support their claims to status" (2000, 1). While we might question this assertion, it is noteworthy that it engages the reader in examining practices of the workplace, observing the challenges to these values encountered by persons at all levels of service.

But, even prior to this preoccupation with self-definition, might we not examine the possibility that what it meant to be a professional, what constituted professionalism, was a fundamental intuition, and perhaps the unarticulated motivation of those who chose the helping occupations? Was it not the focus of study, role models, practice and evaluation?

As I personally reflect on this issue, it occurs to me that noblesse oblige speaks to the essence of professionalism, grounded in a belief in the noble character of the occupation itself. It empowers caregivers as persons who cultivate knowledge-based skills in order to provide service to other persons of intrinsic worth and dignity. While this is a personal viewpoint, I suggest it is shared by most others who select *helping* careers because they want to care for people, and it is most likely the inspiration, motive and energy behind the drive to pursue this work. Is this not what it means to be a human person? And yes, professionalism characterized by altruism, other-regarding values and service worth one's life engagement can be its own reward; caring for others is a legitimate source of self-fulfillment.

> In caring for the other, in helping it grow, I actualize myself. The writer grows in caring for his [her] ideas; the teacher grows in caring for his students; the parent grows in caring for his child. Or, put differently, by using powers like trust, understanding, courage, responsibility, devotion, and honesty I grow also; and I am able to bring such powers into play because my interest is focused on the other (Mayeroff 1971, 30).

The cornerstone of any therapeutic relationship is a presupposition of trust. It explicates, in the language of Ramsey (1970), a canon of loyalty. A central belief in the effectiveness of a helping encounter toward healing of self and other is an implicit trust, communicated through the quality, characteristics and boundaries of that relationship. It presupposes the trustworthiness of the caregiver.

Trust and all it implies is presumed to be provided for and protected by a code of ethics—a code, not as something carried in a pocket or purse, or a graphically designed brochure framed and ritualistically installed in one's office. As a professional code, it is an articulation of the values subscribed to by a service group and held and used by individuals as a point of reference, as a reminder and a standard for self-examination and service appraisal.

Perhaps it need not be noted that we do not live in a perfect world; professional persons are no exception to the common frailties and shortcomings of the rest of humanity. At this time, when professional malpractice within all professions and at all levels of society is visible and public, the greatest challenge might be a process that makes us more sensitized and responsive to the gap between professional ideals, individual behavior and the constraints of the workplace on actual practice.

Persons in helping roles, whether parents, guardians or those in service professions, have promises to keep. Licensure attests to public expectations about what these promises are and is premised on the presumed professional and personal integrity of those expected to keep them. The relationship between helper and client-patient is a fiduciary one.

> To be a professional is to profess the ability to help, and that is fundamentally to embody a promise to those in need of help. While all the usual responsibilities of making and keeping promises hold here, there are crucial differences for the fiduciary relation between professed helper and those in need of help. The professional promises to be the finest he or she is capable of being in the sense of knowledge and technical competence. He or she also promises not only to take care of, but to care for the patient and family—to be candid, sensitive, attentive and never to abandon them (Zaner 1991, 54).

And in accenting the essence of the fiduciary relationship, Zaner makes the point "fiduciary relationship must be understood, not as a form of paternalism, but rather on the model of dialogue" (60).

If we have ever entertained a belief in the willingness and ability of professional persons to adhere to prescribed moral codes and presumed codes of ethics to be the assured moral guardians of professional conduct, we now have to acknowledge the challenge posed by this belief and presumption. Pellegrino et al., referring to what appeared to be an immutable canon in the professions of divinity, law and medicine and presumably fixed for all time, notes, "[f]inally, ethicists have for the first time begun to challenge the canons of professional ethics and practice" (1991, vii). This has been precipitated, according to Pellegrino et al., by a more educated public, alert to the erroneous power of expert knowledge in a technological society, exploitation of medical dilemmas by the media, participative democracy, moral pluralism and the demand for autonomy in decision making affecting our lives. They speak of the collapse of ethical standards and note "without the traditional moral standards by which to judge professional performance, we are all increasingly uneasy in relationships which paradoxically demand the highest degrees of moral integrity" (ix).

Brockett (1997), observing the general public distrust in professional claims to expertise and goodwill, takes the position that ethics education concentrating on rules and regulations is misguided. She proposes "that a reconstruction of ethics education that includes the moral perspectives of trustworthy relationships, re-interpreted for the 21st century, is essential if the professions are to survive as autonomous experts in contemporary society and be seen as trustworthy" (iii).

Brockett argues that the professions have inappropriately assumed a role of power and control over clients by requiring that clients show confidence or *reasonable trust* in professional expertise as the essence of professional-client relationships. She contends that confidence is justified only as a preliminary step separate from the *proper trust* that is necessary in a continuing relationship, if it is to be therapeutic, or where expertise is acknowledged to be limited and outcomes are uncertain. Proper trust is essential to the concept of professionalism which is committed to doing good work for the benefit of others. It can only be given voluntarily and is nurtured by a relationship of *authentic respect* or mutual caring particular to the individuals involved in the relationship. Each of the parties in the relationship has the opportunity to recognize differences of opinion that might affect the decisions taken in the course of working together. When it proves impossible or impractical to practice authentic respect in order to build a relationship of proper trust, it is appropriate to resort to the more formal professional-client relationship of *encounter respect* that is limited to the rules of professional behavior designed to generate confidence. Sadly, as Margaret Brockett noted, it is encounter respect that has become the mantra of professionals rather than authentic respect that is more consistent with professionalism (Pers. com. May 2000).

TRUST AND BOUNDARY VIOLATIONS

No issue has so inflamed the emotional responses of all people, and so traumatized the traditional respectability of health and other helping professionals as boundary violations, particularly sexual misconduct. The issue is neither a new one, nor is it localized geographically or by professional occupation. Media coverage on the devastating consequences to victims, individually and collectively, has placed it on screen in every country. Wherever the abuse occurs, and regardless of who the abusers are, the public breaking-out of this issue, long overdue, has dealt a serious blow to the faith and confidence of people. It has shattered their belief in the moral standards presumed to be the hallmark of those who, by tradition, warranted unquestioned respect—in, some instances, veneration. These include clergy, health care professionals and the guardians of the law—the classical professions of ministry, law and medicine.

In North America, and increasingly on the international scene, most people have in some way been touched and scandalized by accusations of sexual misconduct directed against clergy. J.A. Loftus (1994), a Jesuit psychologist, at one time director of one of the largest treatment centres for priests and religious in North America, provides a handbook for ministers, based on his experience at this centre and on his work with other groups. While his study is based on a specific group, primarily Roman Catholic celibate clergy, his population also includes single and married clergy of other faiths. The findings of his study provide insight into the complexity of sexual misbehavior involving issues ranging from so-called simple indiscretions, reportedly one-time thoughtless mistakes, to cases of long-standing sexual exploitation. While the sexual misbehavior of clergy has its own unique character, conditioned by a sacrosanct position in society, their actions are acts of human persons essentially no different from the rest of us. Insights from the work of Loftus apply as well to other professional groups.

Given the high incidence of sexual boundary violations, a critical issue for all health professions is the rehabilitation of persons with sexually addictive behavior. Richard Irons, MD, an addictionist on the medical staff of the Menninger Clinic in Topeka, Kansas, works with persons with sexual addictions and notes the importance of personal recovery as a condition for professional reentry. With Jennifer Schneider, MD, he authored *The Wounded Healer: Addiction-Sensitive Approach to the Sexually Exploitative Professional* in 1999. Their work highlights the high incidence of sexual misconduct in the helping professionals as a serious violation of power and position. The approximately six to nine percent of helping professionals, who have violated codes of ethics and anonymously indicated having sexual contact with a patient or client at some point in their careers, reveals the frequency of these violations

Breach of Trust, edited by John C. Gonsiorek (1995), addresses breach of trust and sexual exploitation by health care professionals and clergy. It is a comprehensive work, including an extensive reference resource for anyone wishing to pursue this issue. A few observations are relevant here. In the preface, Hannah Lerman noted her *surprise* [italics mine] when, at a women's group she conducted in 1970, she heard a story of a person sexually abused by her previous therapist. Her response to this person became history-in-the-making and, by the 1992 conference, the numbers of persons who shared their stories of abuse had increased and were scattered geographically.

The point to be made here is that violation of trust is not a new phenomenon. In an historical overview in Gonsiorek, Gary Richard Schoener refers to concerns about physician-patient sex in the *Corpus Hippocratum*, a body of medical texts compiled during the fourth and fifth centuries B.C. (1995, 4). Public disclosure and current media attention to boundary violations, with accompanying legal challenges, bring these issues to a level of awareness never known before. This fact attests to the need for a conscientization, appropriate education and attention to the purposefulness of codes of ethical practice, their application and usefulness for inspiring and appraising professional vision and activity. And this, indeed, is happening in many areas.

A brief on-line search shows that a wide range of educational resources is available, for example, the Walk-In Counseling Center, Minneapolis, Minnesota, (www.walkin.org), and a training manual (Milgrom 1992) that, at the time of its printing, had been used over a seven-year period by 125 different human service organizations. As a search of the Internet will also show, nursing associations across the world, in responding to boundary violation issues, are taking a proactive role and have developed extensive information packages and guidelines.

While this movement is timely and long overdue, a more fundamental inquiry into the contextual situations that provide for and allow professional misconduct to occur merits attention. By way of clarification, it must be noted that not all reported cases of misconduct are *sexual* boundary violations.

It seems helpful to be reminded, however, that the climate in which health service is provided, whether in office, agency or institution, has changed over the years. In the past, using nursing as an example, being a professional carried with it rather strict and formal protocols. A *professional person* did not sit in the patient's room, much less the caregiver sit on the side of a patient's bed! Emphasis on therapeutic relationships and the informality that ensued have been a welcome change from the rigidity of these protocols. It must be recognized, however, that the boundary between professional caring and client-patient vulnerability is a very fragile one, and the caregiver, by virtue of his or her role, is in a position of power. When boundary issues are examined, it is often at the juncture of this delicate relationship that, unintentionally and unwittingly, violations occur.

Current media coverage of breaches of trust reveals not only the vulnerability of the patient but also the vulnerability of the caregiver. An ethic of care presumes a knowledge of self, which can anticipate and recognize the boundaries that protect both the caregiver and persons served, and the sensitivity to become aware of when a professional relationship is being transformed into a personal one. An ethic of care should also shape standards of service and the procedures used for the appraisal of relationships in the workplace.

How the Health Care System Structures the Workplace

Is an ethic of care possible in the workplace? Perhaps no words are more familiar to persons in health care today than reform, restructuring, downsizing and cost cutting. The words themselves say something about the dominant thrust of health care planning and service at this time. Questions arise as to whether these well-rationalized attempts to address current problems within the system actually improve the quality of service for patients-clients, and whether the so-called reforms enable caregivers to better use their knowledge and skills, that is, to care. There are positive outcomes throughout the health care system including better access, efficiency and, at least in some situations, better financial control. But there is also evidence of the downside of restructuring. In many instances, caregivers maintain they are unable to care the way they believe they ought to, and pressures in both acute and extended care facilities seem to be increasing this difficulty. These pressures come from a variety of sources, including the restructuring itself, stress and overwork, workload and inadequate staffing in the face of changes in patient profiles and patient care needs.

In *Professionalism, Caring, and Nursing,* Eliot Freidson (1990) examines concepts of professions and professionalization, emphasizing that the theme of caring figures in conceptions of both. In drawing attention to the importance of paying close attention to the institutions that structure caring, he provides a graphic picture of three modes of how to conceive work. These modes of work are the perfectly free labor market, the rational-legal or bureaucratic labor market and the occupationally controlled labor market. Freidson presents these three work modes as *ideal types*, mutually exclusive and hostile to each other. The reader will note how elements of each drive the health system, the combination of all three where they exist and the particular features that dominate the system at one time or another.

According to Freidson, in the perfectly free labor market, the primary criterion is economic cost, a commitment to contain costs and improve efficiency. In the free market, the consumer reigns supreme. "The source of its organization is the aggregate outcome of the unplanned choices of individual consumers who are fully informed about the characteristics of what is being offered for sale and who rationally calculate their material self-interest in making their choices" (on-line, n.p.).

The rational-legal or bureaucratic labor market is

> deliberately organized and planned by a central authority that has decided to produce a set of goods or services whose characteristics it has specified and that has chosen how to produce it. Its executives and staff decide what kinds of tasks must be performed to reach their productive goals, create positions or jobs, hire people to perform them according to their own criteria of necessary qualifications, and establish a hierarchy of supervisory positions to assure that the orders of the executive will be transmitted throughout the organization, and obeyed.... In order to effectively control the work that is done, it attempts to routinize the tasks of its workers so as to minimize the use of discretionary judgment and maximize the use of objective, measurable criteria by which to evaluate them (Ibid.).

The occupationally controlled labor market, as Freidson elaborates, is controlled by specialized workers organized into corporate groups; one of its essential features is collegiality or solidarity: "In the professional labor market the primary interest of the workers is more in the quality of their work than in its reliability or cost. . . . Commitment is to the intrinsic quality of the work for its own sake, with its cost and even its reliability being secondary" (Ibid.). Trust in the competence and integrity of professionals is a central feature of the professional model. It is a "trust that they will not turn their monopoly to their own advantage, that they will care and that they will take care to control both themselves and their colleagues in order to ensure that the public is not victimized" (Ibid.).

It is not difficult to note that the models theoretically drawn by Freidson are mutually exclusive. But neither is it difficult to see the elements of each in the work situation and the particular features that dominate the system. We know persons in health management who commit all their energy to budgetary concerns and improving the financial state of the organization or agency. We are also acquainted with the expertise and energy applied by others to better and more efficient organization within and without the system. Systems are designed and replaced by new ones that claim to be better. And the financial resources used in designing, dismantling and redesigning the system are obviously not available at the point of need—the level of hands-on care.

It is helpful to acknowledge the driving forces behind these realities in health service. Populations have increased, a more educated public knows and expects more from the system, available technologies and equipment consume a greater proportion of available budget, salaries are upgraded to match qualifications and cost of living, labor laws and improving the situation of workers thrust new responsibilities on management. These are only a few of the factors that have influenced the management of health care over the past number of years. Good management, viable systems, sufficient financial and personnel resources are absolutely necessary, but there is a downside to the apparent progress.

In the name of efficiency, responsible use of available resources, avoidance of duplication and a host of other good motives, something has been lost. Perhaps the most disturbing observation is the increasing frustration of nursing over not being understood—from more being demanded of them without the awareness by responsible authorities of the impact of change and restructuring on their ability to provide good nursing care. In many work situations, there is low morale, indifference and, for many, the need to simply get the job done without any personal rewards of fulfillment in doing it well.

In the example of the merger of facilities, denominational identities have been sacrificed, thus eliminating from the health system a strong tradition of value-oriented, faith-inspired service, which for decades crafted a culture of service that is difficult, if not impossible, to replicate. This is not to say that nondenominational, public health care facilities and agencies have not provided compassionate, expert care. But for those denominational facilities that still exist, much energy is spent in justifying their existence and in demonstrating that this mix of identities is an asset to society, not a burden or threat. Is the demise of denominational and other smaller health care organizations a reflection of our societal ethos—bigger is better? And is secularism the only viable option in a *so-called pluralistic society?*

The conclusion of Freidson's paper, referred to previously, is relevant:

> [P]rofessionals should never forget that excessive emphasis on cost and standardization is antithetical to the emphasis on quality and caring discretionary judgment that lies at the heart of their mandate. . . . The caring nurse, no less that the caring physician, must make sure that the institutions in which they work provide the conditions by which they can do so (on-line, n.p.).

THE CALL OF CARE

The vast majority of people in health care services are good persons. They are members of government who commit their energies to juggling limited resources and ever increasing needs, attempting to balance personal, family and political demands of their lives as human beings. They are the CEOs caught in the crunch of the pressures of supply and demand, the invitation to other regarding service, the constraints of market-driven values, constricting budgets and bureaucratic controls. These good people include all those in the front lines of service as well, also attempting to establish equilibrium in their own lives in relationships within marriage and family, and always competing with professional responsibilities, and religious and civic expectations. And, of course, they must all put bread on the table.

The health care system, as is the case with other social and community service organizations, is experiencing an extraordinary crisis. The *Random House College Dictionary* defines crisis as a "condition of instability, as in social, economic or political affairs, leading to a decisive change;" or in a medical context, "the point in the course of a serious disease at which a decisive change occurs, leading to recovery or to death" (s.v. "crisis"). One writer has interpreted the situation in crisis as the experience "of being condemned to the anxious space between the no-longer and the not-yet" (Rowe 1980, 13). These definitions strike a familiar chord for all living through health care reform, restructuring, downsizing and cost cutting. *Chaos* is the word frequently used as an overriding label for the complex dilemmas not easily amenable to understanding and, by their very nature, not open to simple remedies. Economic pressures and bureaucratic structures exert controls over management and operational systems; technology and the demands of a "fix-it" culture complicate the process of decision making at all levels of service.

While granting the reality of moral pluralism, another outstanding issue seems to be the need to cope with moral ambiguity in the workplace. But is this not the call of care in health services as we move into the twenty-first century? As noted previously in this work, health care is a moral enterprise; the health care system a community of persons in relationship. Service is provided not by mathematical calculus and technique, not by the automatic application of the latest and best technological innovations but by negotiation and dialogue in a context of freedom and mutual respect. This is never easy.

But is there evidence of caring within the health care system? Of course there is. And we can find it if we focus on what individuals and groups are doing, and if we concentrate on the evidence this provides. As a patient in hospital following major surgery, I remember, in particular, a nurse coming to my room and, almost apologetically, asking to borrow my flowers! I was delighted to share my beautiful flowers for the celebration of Eucharist in a lounge for a terminally ill patient, his family and friends. This was a celebration over and above the demands of *routine* care, organized in the midst of a very busy unit and planned for one patient among many others who had special needs at this time. It was a healing experience for me in my room to hear this celebration in the background and continues to inspire me as a paradigm case in which caring is supreme. It is one of many such examples.

Susan Phillips and Patricia Benner speak of the importance of sharing caring narratives. "If caring practices are to be noticed, affirmed, and restored, this must happen in the context in which they take place" (1994, vii). In emphasizing the importance of narratives, they continue, "We believe it is essential to recover the vision of what is possible in actual practices today in order to discover the mandates for reshaping our institutional structures, environments, and economics to serve attentive, sustaining, and healing relationships" (vii). What could happen if caregivers were given or took the opportunity to reflect on all the good they do, on all the ways in which they commit their knowledge and skills to make the lives of others better; to cure but always to care? Affirmation begets energy, and if ever persons in health care needed affirmation, they do at this time of crisis and chaos. What happens when caregivers do practice as identifiable professional groups (in the model of Freidson) but, while recognizing the expertise of each, see their service accomplished through partnership and collaboration? I suggest such a climate of care is therapeutic not only for patients and families but also for caregivers themselves. This does occur in some small health care facilities and in specific units of larger health centres.

It is sometimes said, "Nurses don't care any more." Granting the exceptions present among any professional or occupational group, I usually deny the truth of this claim. I suggest it is helpful to reflect even briefly on who the persons are who come to work, for example, in a busy, stressful hospital emergency room on any given day. They are professional people, parents, husbands, wives, sons and daughters, busy persons who respond to demands of family, church and community. Like most busy people, they are often the ones asked to go the extra mile. Under these trying circumstances, nurses do make heroic efforts to respond to the critical needs of persons in their care.

In speaking with professional groups, it has been my experience that probing the experiences nurses bring to the work situation helps to diffuse the guilt many of them feel over not "being caring." Mayeroff's observation is also helpful:

> My life cannot be harmoniously ordered if, for example, there is a basic incompatibility between caring in my work and caring for my family, or between caring for myself and caring for some particular other person. Harmony can tolerate occasional conflicts in priority; there will be times when this caring rather than that comes first. . . . How many carings are required to order our lives fruitfully is, of course, an individual matter, but the number is always small, for we cannot really be devoted to many things at the same time (1971, 57–58).

It is frequently the case, when people realize there are a limited number of persons and projects to which they can commit themselves at any given time, that this understanding itself is sufficient to diffuse the tension, and persons can be energized to care the more. When caregivers are concerned about *not caring*, it is usually not the case that they are not caring, but rather they are in situations where they are *unable to care*, and for legitimate reasons.

Having, in truth, acknowledged the goodness and commitment of the majority of persons involved in all levels of health care, we might still ask if all is well with health care *as a system* itself. I suggest we may not be too far off the mark when we raise a question as to whether or not *as* a system, health care is losing its soul. Is the health care system caught and fixated in the models analyzed by Freidson? Is it not possible that the perfectly free labor market has become its overriding ethos? Has the rational-legal or bureaucratic labor market anesthetized the energy of persons committed to a caring community? Does the occupationally controlled labor market exist as a culture of dominance rather than as a community of persons in collaboration and partnership with all involved in service to others?

Within the quagmire of conflicts and obstructions, impaired by an ethic of materialistic and technological values and impersonal bureaucratic modes of management and practice, the threat to human caring as the prevailing ethic of health service is real. This threat is not only to those served but, as the raison d'être of service itself, it also weakens the empowering attraction of those who select a health care career and nullifies their reason for continuing in the service. Unfortunately, the inability to care and the insurmountable barriers to any hope of improvements in the workplace have moved some committed professional people to opt out of health care and select other careers.

The solutions to the health service crises of our time are neither simple nor easy to come by. The situation in general requires a serious critique that goes beyond mere restructuring or organization and is broader than the responsibility of governing bodies, political or otherwise. The challenge is deeper than better management of what already is and, I suggest, involves a reexamination of how labor-management relations themselves are structured. We might be at the point of asking whether it is time to find an appropriate alternative for collaborative, communal commitments to health care rather than the adversarial model that has served us for so long in the past.

SUMMARY

The conclusion to Mayeroff's work titled, *On Caring,* provides a fitting conclusion to this chapter. To avoid a cumbersome translation of the text, the original wording is left intact on the presumption that Mayeroff's generic use of the word man also includes women.

> Man finds himself by finding his place, and he finds his place by finding appropriate others that need his care and that he needs to care for.

> Through caring and being cared for man experiences himself as part of nature; we are closest to a person or an idea when we help it grow. There is a rock-bottom quality about living the meaning of my life that goes, oddly enough, with greater awareness of life's inexhaustible depths; it is as if life is ordinary and "nothing special" when it is most extraordinary. And although we find a deep-seated intelligibility in life, the last word is with the unfathomable character of existence which, like a pedal point in a piece of music, pervades and colors life (1971, 87).

6

HEALING THROUGH STORY

This chapter is adapted from a presentation given at the Nursing Reflection Conference in Cambridge, England, in June 1998. The poem by Edwina Gateley and the "Cosmic Walk" were choreographed by Dr. Carol Picard, a clinical nurse specialist in mental health-psychiatric nursing who also does professional dance. The presentation was made in an ambience that facilitated quiet meditation, with music and lights marking each point in time with the cosmic walk. You might choose to use this chapter for personal reflection or for group participation. It is a way of expressing care, as well as getting in touch with the sacred mystery of our being in the context of the new understandings of the evolution of the universe. I trust this experience of contemplating the universe will be a sacred and revelatory one.

> We told our stories
> that's all.
> We sat and listened to
> each other
> and heard the journeys
> of each soul.
> We sat in silence
> entering each one's pain and
> sharing each one's joy.
> We heard love's longing
> and the lonely reachings-out
> for love and affirmation.
> We heard of dreams
> shattered.

and visions fled.
Of hopes and laughter
turned stale and dark.
We felt the pain of
isolation and
the bitterness
of death.
But in each brave and
lonely story
God's gentle life
broke through
and we heard music in
the darkness
and smelt flowers in
the void.
We felt the budding
of creation
in the searchings of
each soul
and discerned the beauty
of God's hand in
each muddy, twisted path.
And his voice sang
in each story
His life sprang from
each death.
Our sharing became
one story
of a simple lonely search
for life and hope and
oneness
in a world which sobs
for love.
And we knew that in
our sharing
God's voice with
mighty breath
was saying
love each other and

> take each other's hand.
> For you are one
> though many
> and in each of you
> I live.
> So listen to my story
> and share my pain
> and death.
> Oh, listen to my story
> and rise and live
> with me.
>
> (Edwina Gateley, "The Sharing")

This poem by Edwina Gateley is a fitting opening reflection for the theme of healing through story—the personal story of each of us and the story of the universe, our origin and home. This story of self and universe is really not two stories; it is not about parts, that is, the storyteller, content, reader or listener, humans and otherkind. Its moment is in the telling and the listening, and involves all life. Through a web of interconnectedness, it is one story and its mode of healing is in communion.

The story is a sacred story, bound and bonded by relationship. It is not merely a narration, a recital of events and experiences; it is an interconnection presupposing and birthed in intimacy. The story tells of wandering through caverns of darkness waiting for light, of aimlessly pacing in the desert thirsting for water, of celebrating the earthiness of friendship hoping to fill the empty spaces in the human heart. The sacred story is not something we proclaim for a public audience as a form of entertainment; it is communicated in a sacred space to others in trust. The sharing is often hampered by obstacles and resistance. It delays purposefully for the right person; it hopes for the appropriate time and place; and, within a space of openness, reverence and wonder, it nurtures conditions for growth and healing.

But the story is only story when it is shared; it cannot unfold in isolation. It needs to be communicated to some other. Those who are therapists or who work with patients and families over time know the impact of such initiatives, and the sharing of a life script over and over again. The script may be the same but it is in the telling and in the listening that both client and therapist experience the healing moment.

Just as healing accompanies the unfolding of personal life stories and those of patients-clients and families, so also the healing of our home planet must be attended by its unfolding within the mystery of a universe in an ever-expanding, ever new discovery. We need to be enfolded in the *new story*, not as something we listen to, hear, observe; not as some other from which we are detached. The universe story, from the flaring forth until the present, is about each of us and about all of humankind.

We experience caring and know its meaning in daily life and practice. But, caring as the human mode of being, is not exclusively the call to care for self and other human beings; its call embraces the entire universe. In a sense care for the universe *is* self-care. For as Thomas Clarke, reflecting the thinking of Teilhard de Chardin, notes, "Human beings *are* the universe come to reflective self-awareness" (1991, 29). This is "expanding consciousness" at its highest level.

The planet on which we live is a gloriously magnificent but *one-time endowment*. It has limits and, reading the signs of the time, it seems clear we are at a critical crossroad. Planetary sustainability is at risk to a degree never before experienced. We are involved daily in the destruction of all life forms, in the depletion of soil and other resources, and in the pollution of water and air needed to sustain life. Rachel Carson, in *Silent Spring* (1962), sounded a wake-up call in her assessment of the effects of chemicals—many of them pesticides—on the environment and on all life forms. She documented the destructive effects of chemically treated soil on beneficial species, resulting in an imbalance of the ecosystem. She noted the effects of toxicity on wildlife, on the food chain, and the effects of ingestion on humans. Carson is said to have been both valorized and villanized, but her work led to questioning of the "irresponsibility of an industrialized, technological society toward the natural world" (Carson as cited in McLaughlin 1998, n.p.).

This ecological crisis calls for a commitment to care, not care reduced to slogans and philosophizing but a response empowered by faith in the possibility of positive change and in the ability of all people to make radical choices. It requires nothing less than using whatever personal, political, economic, social and spiritual measures are needed to reverse, or at least slow down, the present course of events. In 1990, Noel Brown, director of the United Nations environmental program, spoke to the universal challenge to care:

> Clearly, this is a vital and auspicious moment for Humanity to reassert our compassion, care and respect for the Earth. Thanks to the perspective provided from space, we are now able to conceive the Planet as a whole and ourselves as a global species with a shared inheritance and a common responsibility. We need now, however, to infuse that vision with a genuine sense of affection, optimism, and hope (Scharper and Cunningham 1993, 23).

The crisis elicits challenge and, as in the case of any family crisis, it is necessary to begin with the story. The universe story is about ourselves; we need to get in touch with its history and with its secrets.

The Universe Story

Brian Swimme, a cosmologist, and Thomas Berry, a cultural historian, provide a strikingly revelatory story in what they include in the title of their 1992 book as a "celebration of the unfolding of the cosmos." In a wonderful reflective and poetic narrative, they recount the unfolding of the universe from the "primordial flaring forth" through the formation of galaxies, supernovas, the emergence of the human species, classical civilizations and what they refer to as the imminent Ecozoic era, a new mode of human-earth relations.

Swimme and Berry speak about the governing themes and the basal intentionality of all existence as governed by *differentiation*—diversity, complexity, variation; *autopoiesis*—subjectivity, self-manifestation, interiority; and *communion*—interrelatedness, interdependence, kinship, mutuality. The cosmogenic principle states that these three characteristics are not derived from some larger theoretical framework but from a post hoc evaluation of evolution itself. They are the cosmological orderings of the creative display of energy everywhere and at any time in the history of the universe (70–79). "Were there no differentiation, the universe would collapse into a homogeneous smudge; were there no subjectivity, the universe would collapse into inert, dead extension; were there no communion, the universe would collapse into isolated singularities of being" (73).

In contemplating the universe, we become aware that each thing, each event is new; each has the capacity for self-manifestation; and all are in relationship to everything else. Repetition, absence of creativity and isolation in the universe are impossibilities. Such insights provide compelling confirmation about who we are as human beings, as unique and unrepeatable individuals; as persons with a claim to a particular identity; and as members of a community always connected and in relationship with all of creation. This fact has profound implications for an ethic of technoscience, particularly at this time when the art of tampering with human life is seen as a great scientific landmark, and when *the triumph of the therapeutic is reflected* in its creation, manipulation and termination.

The universe story is a truly magnificent drama, eliciting responses of reverence and humility, of awe, wonder and always open to surprise. It has been told in many ways and celebrated over time in elaborate rituals. The universe was experienced by early peoples as a sacred place, reverenced by them in a variety of ways. The animal sketches in dwellings of primal peoples demonstrate their lived connection with nonhuman life. Their cultural expressions reveal a close relationship with the cosmos as described by Swimme and Berry as "a life in resonant participation with the rhythms of reality" (1992, 44). And, the authors continue, "For this reason the drum became their primary instrument. The drum was part of the sacred techniques for orchestrating the unity of the human/universe dance" (Ibid.).

While the new science reveals a time-development portrayal of the universe never before known, within modern Western culture something has been lost in the narrative—primarily, a loss of the sacred dimension of all creation. Among the reasons for this catastrophic shift, Thomas Berry notes elsewhere three significant phases accounting for our loss of intimacy with our world:

1. The meeting of early Christian spirituality and Greek humanism formed an anthropocentrism, a worldview that would in the course of centuries so exalt the human as to lose the sense of the human as an integral component of the larger community of existence.

2. Phase two came as a result of the Black Death in Europe (1347 to 1349) that decimated about one-third of the population of Europe. Given the limited knowledge about health, cause, treatment and prevention of disease at that time, people were at a loss to explain the plague and knew much less about how to prevent and treat it. They arrived, consequently, at the erroneous conclusion that the Black Death was a punishment from God; the world was, therefore, evil and wicked. If the world and everyone in it were evil, then all had to come under subjection and domination. The earth had to be subdued. Human beings had likewise to be subdued and in time engaged in many forms of self-inflicted punishment. Humans became separate from the earth, strove to rise above it—to be *in* the world, not *of* the world, an attitude not without long-term devastating effects.

3. The third movement in our loss of intimacy with the natural world, as described by Berry, occurred at the end of the nineteenth century, when "we abandoned our role as an ever-renewing organic agricultural economy in favor of an industrial non-renewing extractive economy" (2000, 130). Shaped by Cartesian philosophy and Newtonian physics, and spurred on by a false optimism over the possibilities of science, a scientific and technological orientation to the world created the *engineers* whose goal was to form a utopian future. Over time, a gradual erosion of the sense of the sacred in one's understanding of the human and the universe resulted, and scientific knowledge was directed to complete domination and control over all earth systems.

The influences of mechanism, dualism, individualism, the privatization of religion and the root metaphor of the machine radically shaped the way of thought and the development of the Western world view. Reason became supreme. Given time, science was to find the solution to all problems. The loss of balance between the scientific, technological and the spiritual, between technoscience and the humanities, crafted the erosion of the sacred dimension of all creation, leading to a crisis never before experienced by the human community.

We now live on a planet where belief in unlimited economic progress, exploitation of air, water, soil and vegetation have stretched to the limit the basic planetary resources needed for human survival. And, according to Swimme and Berry,

> [t]he pathos is that we, even now, are deliberately terminating the most awesome splendor that the planet has yet attained. We are extinguishing the rain forests, the most luxuriant life system of the entire planet, at the rate of an acre each second of the day. Not only here but throughout the planet we are not only extinguishing present forms of life, we are eliminating the conditions for the renewal of life in some of its more elaborate forms (1993, 31).

As far back as 1978, Berry, writing alone, urged us to ponder the meaning of the future in light of:

- energy sources beginning to fail;
- pollution darkening the sky, poisoning the seas;
- tensions between nations and within nations intensifying;
- military methods growing more destructive;
- multitudes of mankind doubling in numbers (In the year 2000, 300 cities over a million will exist; early in the 20th century there were only a dozen such cities); and
- swarming of people toward great urban centres (1).

These concerns are those of every member of the human community and, as Berry notes, we meet as absolute equals to face ultimate tasks as human beings within a human order:

> We have a question of life and death before us, the question however, not merely of physical survival, but of survival in a *human mode of being*, of survival and development into the true splendor of intelligent, affectionate, imaginative persons living in ecstatic enjoyment of the universe about us, in profound interior communion with each other, and with some significant capacities to express ourselves in our arts and sciences, in our music and dance. It is a question of interior richness within our own personalities, of shared understanding and sympathy in our homes and in our families. Beyond this is our extended security and inter-communion with others in an embrace of mind and heart that reaches out to the local community, to the nation, to the larger world of man [woman] to an affectionate concern for all living and non-living beings of earth, and on out to the most distant stars in the heavens. A break, a single destructive antagonism anywhere in the fabric of being is a tear in the heart of every being (1978, 1–2, italics added).

Maguire's recent contribution to a publication devoted to the subject of Christianity and ecology (2000) raises an alarm about the threat of our species to all the foundational elements of life on this planet and about the transformation of the fundamentals of our political economy. The facts are staggering. He notes that:

- less than one percent of the earth's water is usable by humans and unevenly distributed;
- forty-three percent of the earth's vegetated surface is to some degree degraded; it takes from three to twelve thousand years to develop sufficient soil to form productive land;
- the rate of burning fossil fuel will double-glaze the planet by early next century, with unknown consequences;
- four million babies die yearly from diarrhea;
- women constitute seventy percent of the world's 1.3 billion absolute poor, own less than one percent of the world's property and work two-thirds of the world's working hours;
- more than thirty new diseases have been identified since 1973, many of them relating to our new and ecologically dangerous lifestyles;
- overconsumption of the few impoverishes many; and

- new corporate power with increased production and simultaneous increased consumption ravishes the earth and exploits the poor *third-world* countries.

Scharper (1997), complementing these facts, also notes the troubling ingredients of the so-called global ecological crisis. "Acid rain, measurable global warming, rain forest destruction, accelerated species extinction, ozone depletion, a proliferation of toxic waste in our soil, seas and skies are but a handful of the most infamous manifestations of this crisis" (12).

Continued enumeration of threats to the planet at this time can easily immobilize (nothing can be done) or mobilize the global community to care for *mother earth* and, in doing so, to care for ourselves. Such an effort starts with one person, one group, with people who, as von Hildebrand (1953b) describes, have an attitude of *religio*, of reverence for all of creation. Perhaps this begins with an attitude that moves one to mourn: mourn the loss of land, of vegetation, of all living species, of diminishing the resources available to our descendants.

We might define the roots of the crisis of our time as the deprivation of a comprehensive story and of the fixation in the darkness of the reductionist, mechanistic paradigm that has shaped modern Western culture.

> But it seems that something has happened that has
> never happened before: though we know not just
> when, or why, or how, or where.
> Men have left God not for other gods, they say, but
> for no god; and this has never happened before
> That men both deny gods and worship gods, professing
> first Reason,
> And then Money, and Power, and what they call Life,
> or Race, or Dialectic.
> The Church disowned, the tower overthrown, the bells
> upturned, what have we to do

> But stand with empty hands and palms turned upwards
> In an age which advances progressively backwards?
>
> (Eliot 1971, 108).

We need a new story—a new celebratory cosmology that encompasses the universe as community in bondedness, not bondage; that celebrates the earth as subject, not as object to be exploited and consumed. In the great odyssey that is our story, we need to be empowered with a vision of the human person as a participant, not observer, engaged in a web of relationships. We need a new language that replaces the mechanomorphic language of scientific reductionism, a new language about God and about all creation. We need to rethink our understanding of the biblical creation story, to recover the mentality of the image of the human person bonded with the earth as *farmer*, to till and cultivate, not to dominate and subdue (*see* Hiebert 2000).

Rosemary Radford Ruether in a chapter titled, "Ecofeminism: The Challenge to Theology," notes the challenge of ecofeminism to theology in the radicalization that takes place as ecological consciousness is incorporated into feminist theology. Referring to the distortion of the anthropology at the heart of Western thought—the dualisms of soul and body, and the assumptions of the priority and controlling role of male-identified mind over female-identified body—, she notes a correlation between patriarchal domination of the earth with the domination and suppression of women:

> . . .we need to use our special capacities for thought, not to imagine ourselves ruling over others, superior to them, and as escaping our common mortality, but rather to celebrate the wonder of the whole cosmic process and to be the place where this cosmic process comes to celebrative consciousness. We also need to use our capacities to contemplate and understand these processes so that we may harmonize our lives with the life of the whole earth community. This demands a spirituality and ethic of mutual limitation and of reciprocal life-giving nurture, the very opposite of the spirituality of separation and domination (2000, 104).

We are just beginning to intuit the vast implications of the revelations of cosmogenesis, leading us through science to go beyond scientism;

to move from mechanistic mindsets to acknowledgment of mystery beyond the evidence of what is scientifically knowable. Science can go back to the flaring forth of the great fire ball but from where is the fire?

Einstein, with a shamanic quality of imagination and intellectual subtlety, transformed the Newtonian science of his day in his teaching of relativity (*see* Swimme and Berry 1992, 238). And quantum physics, the end result of a reductionist investigation of the elementary constituents of matter, resulted in an understanding that was a surprise twist from a static view of the universe. (*See* Swimme and Berry 1992, 39–45). The universe is now understood not as a fixed container, in which each particle has a fixed address, but rather as a mutually evocative, interconnected, dynamically expanding system. This new knowledge, a new cosmology, presents a challenge but, most importantly, a radically new personal responsibility that we have never before experienced. Perhaps the following anecdote underscores the immediacy of this responsibility.

> The NBC evening news of 28 May 1998 included two items. The first focused on worldwide disturbance over nuclear testing in India and Pakistan. One television image showed the ritual closing of the gate on the border between India and Pakistan. The accompanying commentary referred to decades of political, ethnic and religious rivalry between these two countries; the images portrayed piercing animosity in the eyes of formally attired guards on either side of the gate. The second item reported a new finding by the Hubble Telescope—the discovery of a planet never before seen—two quadrillion miles away in the constellation Taurus, outside our solar system and judged to be larger than Jupiter.

Is it not striking to note that both these events became possible because of the intellectual genius of physicists, of modern achievements in science and technology? In one instance, we have developed the nuclear capacity to destroy the entire planet. In the other, we have advanced the technological capability of piercing the veil into outer space, revealing a magnificent universe in the process of expansion, inviting us to capture a new vision of ourselves in relationship with an interconnected cosmos. The responsibility lies in the choice we have, in a limited period of time, to opt for planetary annihilation or the ecstasy of greater discovery; to save or lose the most magnificent of all planets, the only one we know to date that is capable of producing and maintaining life. Caring, as the human mode of being, calls all professional groups to flesh out a timely response. "For what is at stake is not simply an economic resource, it is the meaning of existence itself. Ultimately it is the survival of the world of the sacred. Once this is gone the world of meaning truly dissolves into ashes" (Swimme and Berry 1993, 31).

The new cosmology aims to draw all persons into a web of relationships with the universe. This requires a radical shift in our psychic awareness as we try to experience ourselves involved in the story, a story within which and, in the context of science, alienation is theoretically impossible. Like all good stories the message is found in symbol and ritual, in its urgency and relevance for our time, opening to our grace and our limitations. It is in the telling and receiving that we own more fully the truth of the story and begin to claim healing. Walking or dancing through the cosmic walk, or even imaging such a wonderful flow of life and life forms from the original flaring forth, can be an experience of awe and wonder. The reader is invited to use this walk in whatever way it leads into the marvelous history of life development over fifteen billion years.

"The Cosmic Walk"

15 billion years ago	The universe was dreamed into being. It contained all the light, energy and potential for everything that would ever come to be, all contained within the miracle of hydrogen.
1 billion years later	This expanding energy began to slow down, cool, differentiate, and all the primal stars and

	galaxies took shape. Stars are made of hydrogen and helium and consume themselves to create the other heavier elements.
4.6 billion years ago	Our mother star in the Milky Way, having consumed herself, collapsed. In the intense energy of that collapse she was transformed into a supernova—exploding her stardust into space and seeding all the new elements that would take shape as the whole body of chemistry.
4.5 billion years ago	That exploding stardust began to slow down, cool and condense into a community of planets around the remnant of the mother star, our sun. Our solar system was born.
4.1 billion years ago	The earth, a privileged planet, cooled and gradually formed an atmosphere, oceans and land mass.
4 billion years ago	Gradually, within the seas, more complex materials began to form, then amino acids and finally proteins. The first simple cells formed and in them the earth awakened into life.
3.9 billion years ago	The earth learned to take nourishment from the sun. Through single cell microbes, she learned to eat sunlight, to "nurse from the sun." Photosynthesis was invented and laid the pattern for all future life forms: that each must receive nourishment from another and give itself in return to become nourishment.
2 billion years ago	The earth's earlier carbon membrane was absorbed, slowly releasing oxygen and forming a new oxygen atmosphere within which all future life would evolve.

1 billion years ago	Life was mysteriously drawn toward union and the first simple-celled organisms began to reproduce sexually. Different strands of genetic memory were combined in their new offspring, opening up infinite new possibilities.
700 million years ago	The first multicellular life forms emerged and creativity expanded rapidly.
510 million years ago	The first fish forms with backbone emerged, protecting the earth's earliest nervous system and the development of her sensory organs.
425 million years ago	The first life forms left the oceans, having developed a membrane within which they could carry their own water. They became the first land plants.
395 million years ago	The mysterious coming and extinction of dinosaurs. The first insects emerged, forming an interdependent community with the land plants.
210 million years ago	The continents shifted, cracked and drifted apart. The oceans were formed.
150 million years ago	The first birds took flight and the earth broke into song.
120 million years ago	The emergence of flowering plants which concentrated their life energy into seed, making protein available for mammals and bringing color and fragrance to earth.
114 million years ago	The first placental mammals emerged, warm-blooded creatures who carry their young within their own bodies and nourish them from their own substance.
40 million years ago	The various orders of mammals are complete.

3.3 million years ago	Current ice ages of earth began, shaping the mountains, valleys, rivers, lakes and streams which formed our present bioregions.
2.6 million years ago	The earliest humanoid types develop, with brains and nervous systems complex enough for the earth to awaken into self-conscious awareness.
40,000 years ago	Modern *homo sapiens* emerged, developing earliest language patterns and occupying Australia and Africa.
20,000 years ago	The flowering of matrilineal societies that involved female deities based on the fertility and abundance of the earth.
10,000 years ago	Humans learned to cultivate plants and domestic animals and settled throughout Asia and the Americas.
5,200 years ago	An age of chronic warfare began, which continues to the present.
5,000 years ago	Megalithic stone structures appear in Europe, Asia and the Americas, marking a transition to warring, male images of the divine.
4,000 years ago	The call of Abraham.
3,200 years ago	The exodus of Israel out of Egypt.
2,500 years ago	The flowering of ethical and spiritual consciousness through the works of Confucius in China and Buddha in India.
2,300 years ago	Classic Mayan civilization flourished in the Americas.
2,000 years ago	Jesus, the Dream of God, brought His message of unity with all people throughout Judea.
400 years ago	The people of Europe invaded and colonized

	other continents, uprooting indigenous people and confiscating their lands and cultures. A period of slave trade and migration was initiated.
200 years ago	A period of intense revolutions, social, scientific and industrial, all of which have shaped our present age.
65 years ago	Humans discovered an expanding universe and the interior depths within atomic structures.
30 years ago (1972)	Humans, on a journey to colonize the moon, turned around and saw the earth as a whole for the first time.

The story continues and, today, all humans can know their common origin with the entire earth community in a single sacred universe. Perhaps it is the beginning of a new world.

I will make a covenant for them on that day,
with the beasts of the field,
With the birds of the air,
and with the things that crawl on the ground.
Bow and sword and war
I will destroy from the land,
and I will let them take their rest in security.
On that day I will respond, says the Lord;
I will respond to the heavens,
and they shall respond to the earth;
The earth shall respond to the grain,
and wine and oil,
and these shall respond to Jezreel.
I will sow him for myself in the land,
And I will have pity on Lo-ruhama [the Unloved].
I will say to Lo-ammi [Not-my-people], *"You are my people,"*
and he shall say, "My God" (Hosea 2: 20, 23-25).

7

EDUCATION AND PRACTICE FOR PROFESSIONAL CARING

Timothy O'Connell, in *Making Disciples: A Handbook of Christian Moral Formation* (1998), shares his experience of many years in teaching moral theology. He was a good teacher; his students did well and were involved in a successful program of studies. For a number of reasons, O'Connell notes, he began to question the impact of his course on students:

> Little by little I came to a painful realization: whatever else I had achieved in those classes, I had not made contact with those levels of the students where they truly lived. I had not touched the metaphors and images out of which they constructed their personal visions of life. I had not brought them to a point where they would (or could) genuinely embrace the moral perspectives of the best of our tradition and make them their own (2).

EDUCATION AND PRACTICE AS TRANSFORMATIVE

That O'Connell's work demonstrates the change that took place in his own teaching is not the issue here. The questions he raises, however, do challenge the illusion we still may have about the degree to which students are actually changed as persons as a result of their learning experiences in health care education and practice. Is it possible we still function with the belief that, as long as we can impart knowledge in a clear, sequential fashion and students can absorb ideas, are able to organize and show a grasp of knowledge in their papers or on written examinations, all is well? The following examples show how this illusion has been borne out in my personal experiences of teaching.

I taught ethics to nursing students in a large tertiary care teaching hospital and did ethics presentations and some rounds in that facility for four years. The course I taught emphasized constitutive moral rules, grounded students in relevant principles and presented all within the grand design of major ethical theories covered in philosophical ethics of that time. Yes, case studies were included and, in collaboration with other teaching faculty, a major effort was made to integrate ethics content with clinical teaching and practice at various levels of the program. The teaching method evolved from workshops and consultation with faculty and was thought to be a *good* way of presenting ethics content. The questions remain: Did students and faculty as well come out of their experience better persons? Did the experience enable them to attain an appreciable level of moral maturity with at least the basic essentials for personally and professionally living up to the moral standards around which the program attempted to engage them? Were our presumptions that, in fact, the experience did have such a transformative impact ill-founded? There is no doubt good was accomplished. Whether, in the words of O'Connell, students and faculty alike genuinely embraced the moral perspectives of the program and made them their own is open to question.

Another personal experience involved an incident a few years earlier with a student who had come to my office for a matter that was, as I recall, not of particular importance. An issue arose, however, from a casual comment about a minigroup research project in which she was engaged as a requirement for a course in another department of the university. This senior student had taken a full-year course in ethics in her third year and was completing a nursing program that implicitly and explicitly integrated the Christian human values thought to be foundational in the curriculum. She was a very intelligent girl, a good student, and could be seen as a person of moral integrity. But this mini-, innocent research project, intended to measure a specific behavior of students—selected at random on campus and invited to participate—, involved a violation of moral rules that the student failed to recognize. These included violations of trust, truth-telling and promise-keeping, all touching the issue of respect for students invited for the study. The focus of the project was on testing a specific behavior; ethical issues involved in the method of doing so were missed. The student was disturbed when questions about the procedure brought these issues to her attention, indicating she was not morally indifferent to them, and she was permitted to use a written presentation as a substitute for the project.

This brief experience was a powerful *teachable moment* through which the student internalized ethical values in a manner not accomplished during formal teaching sessions. The question still remains: Did formal course requirements, including ethics, intensive study, reading and writing of papers and examinations and the context of the curriculum itself miss something of paramount importance in the philosophy of this program, if not fail to achieve its intended goals? Admittedly, many factors not addressed here are involved in teaching, learning, the internalization of values and in the formal protocols for research. The issue bears more on the question of teaching and learning as transformative.

In the experience of most educators, when priority is given to cognitive learning, questions around commitment to holistic development of both teachers and students still prevail, even though health care programs appear to be holistic and look very different. We have come a long way from dependency on formal educational taxonomies as tools for appraising achievement. Nonetheless, it is not always clear who and what we are evaluating, particularly if there is a split between our understanding of what it means to be a professional and what it means to be a human person with a specific professional identity.

Is education for life and living, for the development of the whole person, for the formation of persons for the professions or is it exclusively geared to the preparation of the practitioner with the knowledge and tools required to do a *good job*? Is the grand design of educational programs, whatever they are—but specifically for persons being prepared for service in the health professions—, limited by the knowledge, skills and the practice boundaries determined by discrete professional roles? Or is it formative for living at a time that requires expanded vision, a firing of the imagination and an openness to an entire new way of thinking in a culture that can no longer be supported or held together by the technoscience of a mechanism paradigm? As culture, emerging from the era of modernism, awakening to the need for a shift in thinking, seeking a new orientation to personal, family and global values, we are invited and challenged to think about the formidable responsibility education has at all levels for shaping the future. Education has to be about transformation and has to presume the professional and the personal are inseparable.

I suggest it is helpful to take a brief tour through the dominant features of Western culture that have shaped our way of thinking about ourselves and our world and, despite claims to the contrary, still influence lifestyle and social institutions as we enter this twenty-first century. This is particularly relevant for an appraisal of the philosophy and political structure of health care.

HEALTH SERVICES IN A HISTORICAL CONTEXT

Health care as personal-communal service to persons in need has solid historical roots in the Hebrew and Christian traditions. For the Hebrews, who embraced a theocentric philosophy, life was not separated into religious and secular. Service to neighbor, particularly the sick, was a normal expression of their faith, and their religious and social identity. As Donahue notes,

> Ancient Jews believed that all men should have access to medical care, regardless of their social status. With an emphasis on human brotherhood and social justice, the duties of hospitality to the stranger and relief for widows, orphans, the aged, and the poor were constantly urged as righteous. Visiting the sick was a prominent feature of everyday life and a designated duty (1985, 57).

Their houses for strangers, *xenodochia*, are precursors of the modern inn and the modern hospital.

The early Christians likewise considered care of the sick as an expression of their way of life, taking inspiration from the life of Jesus of Nazareth, and the way of being with others that he modeled, as recorded in the Christian scriptures. Early hospices and, later in monasteries, *Christ Rooms* provided a sacred space where the sick and injured were welcomed and cared for. Over time, the commitment of religious orders of men and women to the care of the sick became a natural expression of the Christian mission's emphasis on the spiritual and corporal works of mercy. Fired by this same sense of mission, health care ministry in home and hospital expanded throughout Christianity up to our modern denominational health care institutions.

The cultural seismic shift, spurred on by modernism in the West, antireligious movements and the secular philosophies of our own day, radically shifted the ethos of Western society. This shift from a *theocentric-Christocentric* worldview *to* one of so-called pluralism split the public and private spheres of life, removing the formal recognition of religious witness from public affairs and, in some instances, by political oppression, forced it to the underground.

This is not to say that everything of the past was good and that abuses of different kinds did not flaw the mosaic of Christianity at many levels in its long history. But, from the sixteenth century on, the gradual impact of Cartesian dualism, of the mechanistic thrust of liberalism, scientific Marxism, and the idolatry and religion of progress based on reason alone, dealt a death blow to the foundations of human personal and societal moral life. But the human spirit is hard to crush and the hunger and search for spirituality, for an integral humanism beyond the narrow borders of a mechanistic metaphor, challenged the false optimism grounded in scientism and the supremacy of reason. (*See* Sorokin 1942; Solzhenitsyn 1978; Winter 1981; Capra 1982; Smith 1982; Baum 1985; Holland 1987; Toulmin 1990; Tarnas 1991; Wilbur 1996; Lakeland 1997).

Gibson Winter, challenging the machine as root metaphor of modern culture, speaks of the artistic metaphor as an alternative, expressing the need to live by an artistic, relational paradigm to make visible the invisible through artistic representation. He asserts this artistic, relational paradigm holds some promise of transcending the incoherence and anarchy of the mechanistic age. Speaking of the artistic process, he identifies this "one principle option for the contemporary Westernized world: to accept gratefully its creative powers; to comprehend how these powers may be modes of attunement to nature and knowledge rather than modes of domination and exploitation" (1981, 11). Winter continues to say, "[W]e depend upon such metaphoric power to open a horizon of possibilities, with a vision to judge and liberate our age" (24). The artistic metaphor expresses the need to live by an artistic, relational paradigm, a way of living that is bound by dialogue and creativity. In response to a letter that focused on how his ideas on the artistic metaphor reflect the recovery of nursing's traditional charism of human care, Winter notes that the "more creative, caring understanding of the human being radically shifts the paradigm," that is, from mechanistic to artistic metaphor (pers. com. 27 March 1993).

This brief commentary is an overly simplistic translation of the centuries of cultural evolution of Western civilization that *transformed* the values, the way of perceiving self and others, attitudes toward work and living, relationships with God, with church and with neighbor. The point being made is that it was a *transformative* process that shaped modernism, with its dominant mechanistic influence nurtured by a philosophical dualism and a belief in the supremacy of science to create unlimited progress. In so doing, it planted the seeds for failure that we now experience globally. In this postmodern age, might we hope for a transformative seismic shift of a different kind? Who do we want to be as persons? How do we want to be as family and community? How would we like health care to be fashioned? What are our hopes for this planet on which we live?

Transformative Learning: A Global Perspective

Professor Edmund O'Sullivan, coordinator of the Transformative Learning Centre, Ontario Institute for Studies on Education (OISE),

University of Toronto, published a timely work, *Transformative Learning: Educational Vision for the 21st Century* (1999). With a foreword by Thomas Berry, his book is described by Stephen Dunn, director, Elliot Allen Institute for Ecology and Theology in Toronto, as a text of "rare discernment in a time of turbulent change." O'Sullivan's work is not a how-to of educational reform. But, in a scholarly, comprehensive style, he focuses on what he believes is formatively appropriate for the emerging culture of our time. He speaks to the urgency for structuring education within a comprehensive cosmology, with educational programming capable of engendering what he calls a planetary vision. Critiquing the functional appropriateness of the dominant vision of the global marketplace, he indicates what he considers to be the currents that must be part of an "emergent vision of transformative-ecozoic education" (6). I suggest the reader will find *Transformative Learning*, capturing caring as the human mode of being in a universal sense, a rich resource, insightful and thought-provoking. It provides a context for meaning at this time of chaotic transition—a time replete with possibilities for a future not yet determined.

Reflecting on O'Sullivan's vision, I could not help but think about the Summit of the Americas recently held in Quebec, Canada, as well as those previously convened in other countries. I wondered to what extent the powerful global marketplace vision overrides the countervision he and others are vigorously making through appeals, submissions and protests that seek the global values of justice, concern for the poor, gender equality, environmental protection and global sustainability. And, of course, all these values are intimately in tandem with commitment to the health of persons and communities the world over.

Jean Watson (1999) in her most recent work, *Postmodern Nursing and Beyond*, proposes a "postmodern, transpersonal caring-healing model" echoing the artistic metaphor of Winter, while also encompassing O'Sullivan's cosmological approach. It explicates the following premises that, in their significance for this work, I quote in full:

- There is an expanded view of the person and what it means to be human—fully embodied, but more than body physical; an embodied spirit; a transpersonal, transcendent, evolving consciousness; unity

of mindbodyspirit; person-nature-universe as oneness, connected.
- Acknowledgment of the human-environment energy field—life energy field and universal field of consciousness; universal mind (in Teilhard de Chardin and Bohm's sense of *mind*).
- Positing of consciousness as energy; caring-healing consciousness becomes primary for the caring-healing practitioner.
- Caring potentiates healing, wholeness.
- Caring-healing modalities (sacred feminine archetype of nursing) have been excluded from nursing and health systems; their development and reintroduction are essential for postmodern, transpersonal, caring-healing models and transformation.
- Caring-healing processes and relationships are considered sacred.
- Unitary consciousness as the worldview and cosmology, i.e. viewing the connectedness of all.
- Caring as a moral imperative to human and planetary survival.
- Caring as a converging global agenda for nursing and society alike (129).

In the remainder of her work, Watson provides creative ideas that flesh out the previous premises, and she provides confirmation of them through suggested practices. Watson's vision does not warrant further commentary other than to express its synchronicity with the thinking of writers like Edmund O'Sullivan, and its coherence with the focus attempted in this work on *caring as the human mode of being*. It is appropriate here, however, to express my indebtedness to Jean Watson as a person who was influential in the first stages of my work on caring and who is a moving source of inspiration as I continue to develop a conceptualization of human caring that always remains unfinished.

Transformative Learning: Caring as Response to Value

The affirmation of caring as the human mode of being is a presupposition for all the activities designed to develop the capacity to care professionally. The professional development of this capacity to care is presumed to be possible through a variety of approaches, developed through the creativity of teachers and students and through uniquely designed basic and continuing educational programs. In this process, an environment where caring models are visible is imperative. In the late 1980s, at the invitation of Dr. Anne Boykin, I had the privilege of spending a day with nursing faculty and students at Florida Atlantic University (FAU). In its commitment to ensuring the visibility of human caring as the root and foundation of nursing education and practice at all levels, FAU provides distinguished leadership and demonstration through its philosophy and models of learning. (The selected writings of Parker and Barry [1999], Boykin and Parker [1997] and Boykin and Schoenhofer [2001] are referenced in this chapter.)

The following reflections relate specifically to caring as responsivity—caring as response to value, based on the work of Dietrich von Hildebrand (1953a) used in previous research on the implications of a theory of value for nursing curriculum (Roach 1970).

Von Hildebrand refers to value as an ultimate datum, a self-evident fact of experience that has importance. Differing from a theory of value as subjective—something has value because I value it—it does not seek further proof other than that it is: it is self-evident. Considered in the objective sense, values are there whether or not I value them. The value is not in my feeling or self-satisfaction. This is not to say that feelings are irrelevant, that self-satisfaction is unimportant or is not experienced when I care for or about someone, something or some project. But the value about or for which I care is not in my self-satisfaction per se but in that for which I care.

According to von Hildebrand, caring as responsivity affirms values that fall into different categories. These encompass ontological values—those according to the nature of the object, for example, the sacredness of human life; the preciousness of the human being; the inherent dignity of each patient; and qualitative values—classified into different value domains such as esthetics, spiritual, cognitive, moral, political and economic. He notes a hierarchy between the ontological and qualitative categories, between the qualitative value

125

domains and the specific values within each domain. For example, it seems logical to assert that the sacredness of human life is of a higher order than intellectual acuteness; that moral values are of a higher order than the value of individual economic success; and that the well-being of a community has priority over an individual's right to engage in actions that cause harm to other individuals or groups.

As responsivity, caring is a response to a value—value in myself, in the project I undertake, in the human beings with whom I minister, in the persons with whom I live or relate to professionally. The value is in the person, thing and project; in goodness, virtue, and so on, as the important-in-itself. The latter is intrinsically and autonomously important.

The value response is essentially different from a response motivated by the subjectively satisfying. When the response is motivated by the subjectively satisfying, the object is appropriated and sacrificed to the person responding. Von Hildebrand asserts:

> The value response, on the other hand, is characterized by an element of respect for the good, an interest in its integrity and existence as such, a giving of ourselves to it instead of a consuming of it. Even in cases where a value response aims at the fruition of a good endowed with value, the element of self-donation and interest in preserving its ontological dignity and integrity dominate the entire situation (1953a, 216).

One of the decisive marks of the value response, then, is its character of self-abandonment. It is a break from self-centredness to the important-in-itself. Interest in the subject is nourished by the intrinsic goodness of the object. Value response is essentially a conforming to the value. This self-abandonment implies a transcendence that, according to von Hildebrand, is opposed "not only to an imminent, blind teleology, but also to a self-imprisonment" (Ibid., 217). It is important to emphasize here that self-abandonment and self-transcendence, as used by von Hildebrand, are terms not equivalent to self-depreciation or the kind of self-denial motivated by low self-esteem or neglect of self. He makes much of the notion of transcendence as representing one's uniqueness as a personal being. It "lights up his [her] character as an image of God" (217). He continues:

> The difference between an appetite or an urge and a value response clearly reveals the essential immanence of the first and the

transcendence of the second.... There is a yawning abyss between the nurse who ministers to us with care because she wants to appease her motherly instincts and the nurse who surrounds us with all possible attention and care because of her love of neighbor and her real sympathy for our suffering and needs (1953a, 220).

One might add, it is probable each source of motivation is part of the nurse's total person response. There is personal fulfillment in caring for others, but von Hildebrand asserts that one's nature is "ordained to transcend itself and to be capable of real self-donation" (Ibid., 222). This, too, is self-fulfillment.

Another mark of the value response is its relationship to call. As a human being, I am drawn to the good, the beautiful, the important-in-itself. In this sense, being drawn is a response to a call: the good and the beautiful call me. The objective value calls forth a response that is care; care awaits the call of the important-in-itself. The response and the call are reciprocal.

B. Somfai (pers. com. 1984) believes a further consideration involves the relationship between caring and dependency. Care or the act of caring is a response to a fundamental characteristic of human existence, a transcendental property that is dependency. The term dependency describes the fact that, as human beings, we come into existence through the efforts of someone else. We owe not only our existence to the care of others but becoming what we are is also the result of the loving, protective care of parents, relatives, family and community. Care stands in dialectical relationship with dependency.

Ordinarily, care is exercised by those immediately connected or involved with us—family members, friends and relatives. Care is also exercised by members of society whether by office or by profession—nurses, physicians, lawyers or teachers. This transcendental character of dependence and the corresponding universal need for care is expressed most dramatically, however, in critical situations where the traditional bonds and boundaries of care break down. Consider, for example, our spontaneous reaction as we watch the evening news where violence is the main item on the agenda. Note our affective response to what we perceive to be inhuman (absence of care) in events that touch the personal and family lives of people in our own communities and all over the world; the desperate plight of the poor and homeless; the daily destruction of life systems on our planet. The universal need for care manifests itself in critical situations, in peak experiences, when our dependence on others and on the earth itself affects our very growth, development and even survival. Caring is a response to dependency.

Willard Gaylin discusses the relationship between caring and dependency from the perspective of "the utter helplessness of human infants, and their total incapacity to survive without the ministrations of the adult members of the community" (1979, 36). He uses dependency as a vehicle for "exploring, substantiating, and elucidating the caring nature of the human being" (Ibid.). In his analysis of the human situation, in contrast to animal behavior, Gaylin postulates that

> . . . no species so designed could have survived the hundreds of thousands of years from its inception to a point of organized civilization where such codes of conduct might have been imposed and transmitted via cultural heritage, unless there had been from the beginning an innate genetic response of caring and loving for the helpless newborn (41).

This awareness of helplessness and lovability as power, and the potential of both to elicit care, is learned in infancy. That it is learned is profoundly important in shaping a model of relationships for adult life. As Gaylin notes, "The 'power' of helplessness fuses with the 'power' of lovability to become an essential part of the complicated dependency lessons that the infant will almost inevitably carry into his adult life" (Ibid.).

AFFECTIVE RESPONSE AND "BEING AFFECTED"

The distinction von Hildebrand makes between the affective response and being affected has important pedagogical significance, particularly where the calling forth of the caring capacity is at the core of health professional learning and practice. His discussion of intentional and unintentional experience is relevant to reflections on caring as virtuous action. Intentional experiences refer to the conscious, rational relationship between the person and an object. In contrast, unintentional experiences refer to mere states such as tiredness, cheerfulness, sadness and those trends in our nature that represent a blind push toward something. The affective response is ordinarily preceded by the experience of being affected, and this presupposes knowledge. As von Hildebrand puts it: ". . . when the beauty of noble music or the nobility of a moral act moves us, a grasp of the object and a perception of its value are presupposed. Moreover, there exists a meaningful intelligible relationship between the object affecting us and the effect created in our soul" (1953a, 208). Being affected, having a centripetal character (the object bestows something on me) differs from the affective response with its centrifugal character (I, by my response, impart something to the object). Nevertheless, being affected is closely related to and ordinarily precedes the affective response.

A truly human response to value calls into operation the spiritual power of affectivity, which, in cooperation with the intellect, responds with joy, esteem, contempt, enthusiasm, veneration, love or compassion. In such a response, there is an inner, spiritual, meaningful and intentional relationship between the person and the object in contrast to that of a mere feeling state.

The insights of von Hildebrand contribute to an understanding of what is involved in caring as responsivity, caring as a response to value as the important-in-itself, caring as intentional, habitual, virtuous activity. Von Hildebrand, in *The New Tower of Babel* (1953b), refers to it as the response of a person pervaded by an attitude of religio. It is a life framed by obligations; a life "pervaded by the consciousness that every good possessing an authentic value calls for an adequate response" (50). This is the responsivity entailed in human caring, in caring expressed through virtuous acts.

The major question posed by T.E. O'Connell about the work cited previously is relevant here: How can we so design educational experiences and the practice space so that they enable teachers, students and practitioners alike to perceive caring as a value in itself, to *value caring as an ontological value having qualitative expressions in everyday practice*? How can we turn objective values (honesty is a moral good) into subjective values (I choose to be honest) enabling individuals to make them their own? (*See* O'Connell 1998, 58). This question is further addressed in reflections on caring as virtuous activity.

Transformative Learning: Caring as Virtuous Action

In a previous chapter, attention was given to virtue ethics. The Greek word for virtue, *arete*, is interpreted as an excellence that denotes the power of something to fulfill its function. "Virtue is something within human nature that inclines us to choose those acts which fulfill our nature as human beings" (Pellegrino and Thomasma 1996, 20). Theological reflection modifies this sense of virtue as *natural* with the insight that supernatural virtues are free gifts of God, which dispose us to direct our lives according to our identity and human destiny. In the context of this work and the underlying presuppositions about the human person as body-mind-spirit unity, the natural and supernatural are not compartmentalized into separate entities but expressive of the identity of the person as made in God's image.

Caring is seen as the virtue at the heart of who we are as human persons and as the core value that inspires, directs and sustains the identity of all engaged in the service of others. I suggest we can assert that caring as virtue, using the words of O'Connell, based on "the intrinsic, nonnegotiable dignity of human persons . . . not rooted in the person's intelligence or utility or beauty or productivity, but rather in [his, her] very created reality" (1998, 25, 26).

TRANSFORMATIVE LEARNING: PRACTICE OF SIX CS

Considerable attention has been given in this work to the ontical expression of human caring as interpreted through the *SIX Cs of compassion, competence, confidence, conscience, commitment and comportment.* It is noted that these are not mutually exclusive but represent a sufficient degree of specificity to enable us to better understand caring in its various ways of being with others. It is helpful to note the specific values implicit and explicit in each of them and the virtuous actions that are their mode of expression.

Explicit values are inherent in the expression of *compassion,* a way of entering into the experience of the other as person of nonnegotiable, intrinsic worth, beauty and dignity; as neighbor suffering and in need; as individual experiencing the pain of trauma, loss, isolation and sorrow; as human beings and communities encountering explicitly the dis-harmony, dis-ease and dis-integration characteristic of the human condition itself. The acquisition of *competence* is the caring person's way of ensuring that he or she is able to provide the highest quality of service that a specific role or responsibility requires. It involves years of preparation and arduous practice, and disciplined effort along with the compensations and fulfillment that it brings. The caring person strives to acquire the personal and professional qualities that inspire trust (*confidence*) in relationships that are difficult, even at times repulsive, as well as in relationships that are enjoyable and gratifying. The caring professional endeavors to develop a fine-tuned *conscience*, responsive to the moral-ethical in teaching and practice, having basic knowledge and skill, while at the same time knowing when and where to seek consultation. The attribute of *commitment* is formative for professional persons who internalize accountability with responsibility and strive to achieve a balance between care for self, for family-significant others and service demands. The sixth C, *comportment,* speaks to the importance of maintaining harmony between beliefs about the intrinsic dignity of self and others, and the manner in which the person comports his-/herself as a professional caregiver.

The explication of values inherent in the SIX Cs and further research on the essence of human caring, as expressed in these and other attributes as virtuous activity, could be an interesting challenge for researchers. Such research, along with identification of already published studies on how such virtuous activity is taught, learned and practiced, would be a most welcome contribution to health care literature. But to undertake such a project, which would include philosophical, theological and other resources, is beyond the scope of this revision and not possible for the writer at this time.

A concluding observation might be helpful. However we may think about or define virtue, it is important to note that virtue can be understood purely as a natural capacity—the capacity to care is an expression of one's humanity that needs to be called forth, nurtured and expressed. But virtue is also a supernatural gift that we do not acquire through our own efforts. Speaking of compassion, Nouwen insists that it is "not a skill we can master by arduous training, years of study, or careful supervision.... Compassion is a divine gift and not a result of systematic study or effort.... It is the revelation of God's divine spirit in us" (1980, 132; *see also* Nouwen et al. 1983). I believe we can teach and learn the skills that build and enhance caring relationships and practice so we become virtuous practitioners through intentional habit formation. We also pray for this gift.

It is important to recognize that the SIX Cs are presented in this work as ideals to which we aspire. As wounded healers, we are called to care for ourselves through the same qualities of compassion we hope to extend to others. For persons in health care roles, it is not easy to believe one needs to be cared for, since it seems easier to give than to receive. To receive care is to recognize our own vulnerability, our own limitations. But the peaceful acceptance of limitation is also a gift that has to be received and accepted. In the experience of the writer, it is the invitation to respond gently toward the experience of the gap between the words spoken and written, and the quality of everyday living. Tacit acceptance of the ideals to which we aspire is not always accompanied by the actual practice of the virtues they embrace; this is the work of a lifetime.

Transformative Learning: Reflective and Contemplative Practice

Donald A. Schon's seminal work, *The Reflective Practitioner*, gave impetus to writing and discourse on reflective practice in educational and other disciplines. In the later *Educating the Reflective Practitioner* (1987), he shows how professional schools might use reflective practice to prepare students to approach difficult situations with skill, confidence and care. Both the nursing and medical professions have utilized a variety of teaching methods to develop the reflective capacities of students, with the expectation of creating a practice environment that empowers learners to enter into their own experience in a way that enhances the quality of their care of patients.

Dawn Freshwater, reporting on the student nurse's experience of reflective practice, observes that it provides a way "for caring individuals to explore and confront their own caring beliefs and how these beliefs are executed in practice" (1999, 29). She adds further, "reflection is not just about gaining access to caring beliefs and contradictions through retrospection, but it is also about transforming self and thereby caring in practice" (Ibid.). Christopher Johns, University of Luton, applying reflective practice in his research and practice over the past several years, has solidified its themes through a succession of reflective practice conferences and his own writing. The following is from the abstract of his 1997 study:

> Guided reflection is a developmental process to enable and empower practitioners [either as individuals or in small groups] to learn through reflection upon lived experience with the intention of realizing caring. Guided reflection is also a collaborative research process, whereby the educator/researcher and practitioner can understand the contextual nature of desirable practice and the factors that limit achieving this practice (33).

Transforming Nursing through Reflective Practice, edited by Johns and Freshwater (1998), covers the story of a group of people who came together after the Third Reflective Practice Conference in

1996 at Robinson College, Cambridge, England. It is a comprehensive resource with the impressive authorship of twenty contributors who presented papers at this conference.

Lynn Wagner (1999, 2000), explores poetry as narrative—the transformative nature of transpersonal poetic reflections—and points to the power of reflective practice for personal and aesthetic knowing. In her writings, she provides several examples of poetic stories and notes how they "fabricate a mosaic of images, a tapestry of wisdom and understanding about the unique and universal aspects of living and dying" (2000, 7).

INTERNATIONAL ASSOCIATION FOR HUMAN CARING (IAHC)

In 1978, the First National Caring Research Conference was convened and hosted by Dr. Madeleine Leininger at the University of Utah. It highlighted the "initial and continuing concern of the conference as—identifying the philosophical, epistemological, and professional dimensions of caring to advance the body of caring knowledge" (Gaut 1993, n.p.). From sixteen participants at the first conference, the association expanded its boundaries to include international membership and with annual conferences in different countries such as the United States, Australia, Canada, Finland and Scotland. IAHC is a forum for administrators, deans, educators, researchers and practitioners committed to the centrality of caring in nursing and the research, education methods and practice that keep it visible in health care. Presentations from the IAHC Conferences have been published as volumes from 1981 to 1995, and from 1997 to the present in the *International Journal for Human Caring*, published quarterly.

Reference in this work to the singular importance of the initiatives and scholarship of IAHC is made because of my involvement with the association over the past number of years. But caring in nursing has also been the focus of many others who, by their leadership, scholarship and practice, continue to keep caring at the centre of their professional commitments. The writings of these leaders are cited elsewhere, but special mention needs to be accorded here to Patricia Benner, a nurse educator, practitioner, lecturer and researcher who has both challenged and inspired the profession internationally.

REFLECTIVE OR CONTEMPLATIVE PRACTITIONER

John Miller, in *The Contemplative Practitioner*, while acknowledging the importance of Schon's work, asserts there is something missing. In his interpretation of reflective practice, Miller claims that by itself it retains a dualistic concept of reality—subject reflecting on the object—that ends up with a "fragmented and compartmentalized approach to life" (1994, vii). He believes that work and daily life can be enhanced by the contemplative life which engages one in a manner that restores the whole and taps a deeper energy within and which can bring joy and purpose to daily experience. I suggest it may not be a question of either/or but of both/and.

Miller's book is a valuable resource for persons who seek the contemplative dimension of everyday life. It is a practical and insightful guide for those who wish to explore the place of study and the practice of contemplation in education for the professions. Teaching administrators and teachers at the graduate level in education at OISE, Miller offers two courses—the Holistic Curriculum and the Teacher as Contemplative Practitioner—in which students are required to do some form of meditation. In his own words:

> The requirement is based on the premise that teaching should come from the Self rather than the ego. Ego-based teaching ultimately reinforces our sense of separateness and suffering. I emphasize that when we teach from the Self, we gradually experience more moments of communion with our students. . . . Holistic education can be defined in many ways. One definition I like is simply the release of the human heart. Meditation is fundamental to that release (1994, 122).

I am inclined to believe that, if Miller, Johns, Freshwater and others came together in dialogue, the differences in perceptions of the reflective and contemplative practitioner would not be too striking. I suggest, however, that contemplation is a foundation for reflective practice.

Holistic education has been at the heart of education for the health professions for many years. Education for health services, by its very nature, is experiential. And the curriculum in nursing schools and in medical education, as well, has been designed so that students encounter the real life health needs of people shaped by the situations that bear on their personal, family and community lives. Students enter health care careers confronted by the concerns of people struggling under the burdens of economic and social pressures, poverty and homelessness, victims and sometimes perpetrators of violence. Outpatient and emergency departments, not only of large inner-city teaching hospitals but also smaller community hospitals, carry a patient and family population marked in varying degrees by the above stresses. The nature and complexity of crises experienced by patients and families seeking health care today are very different to what they were even a few decades ago. And students themselves come out of family and community situations in marked contrast to the more stable home and school environments enjoyed by their predecessors fifty years ago.

The entrance to professional programs in health services in the past presupposed a disposition toward a lifetime service to others; the formative process exacted total commitment to study and, in retrospect, some would claim inhumane practice-service expectations. Nurse *training* was strongly militaristic in most cases and, in Roman Catholic institutions, often structured along the model of religious novitiate formation programs. This was not all bad but cannot be defended in a society that has changed radically toward a greater appreciation of personal autonomy, with many more options for career choice, all encouraged by an educational sophistication that both challenges the old and shapes the new. Education at all levels of society is radically different in 2002 from what it was in the mid-twentieth century and, in both substance and opportunity, carries with it many benefits.

The goals of health care—care of the sick and disabled, promotion of health, prevention of disease and illness in facilities, family and community—have not essentially changed. Given the health profile of society even in small designated neighborhoods, the context within which health care is provided, the characteristics of persons who enter health professional careers, however, make unique demands on educators and students alike. Paraphrasing O'Connell, we might still ask if we are making contact with students at the levels where they truly live. Are we touching the metaphors and images out of which they construct their personal visions of life? Are the philosophical basis of health education, teaching and learning methods founded on a vision that aspires to and at least allows for the formation of students for a virtuous life in caring for self and others?

Summary

This chapter was meant simply to raise issues, not to propose solutions. But the questions raised by O'Connell and the examples of preparation of both reflective and contemplative practitioners are moving us in a direction of positive change. Actually to assume and acquire the identity of professionally caring persons is really to aspire essentially to be loving persons. And I insist caregivers themselves must be cared for, the environment within which they practice must enable them to care and their lives as professionals must somehow be integrated with who they are and wish to be as human persons. I conclude with a kind of *bottom line* statement from Sheila Cassidy:

> More than anything I have discovered that the world is not divided into the sick and those who care for them, but that we are all wounded and that we all contain within our hearts that love which is for the healing of nations. What we lack is the courage to start giving it away (1988, 3).

EPILOGUE

In the "Prologue," I cited a suggestion from Mary Lou Kownacki that "we try to imagine how different life would be if we all recognized and reveled in the present, in the common, as sacrament" (1996, 7). *Sacrament* says much about what this work is about. It is not an ordinary word but a symbol, a sign, a mystery and a metaphor. Sacrament is an encounter, a life ritual, a sign, a mystery and an instrument of the holy in our midst. Sacraments always involve community experienced in distinct forms in different cultures and faith traditions.

The s*even sacraments* of the Roman Catholic Church solemnize significant touchstones in the lifespan of individuals and communities. They ritualize the mysteries of birth and rites of initiation, the seal of identity and membership in the Christian community through anointing with oil and laying on of hands. In union with the Lord of life, they celebrate community through feast and banquet, feeding with Word and Eucharist. They enact moments of healing, forgiveness and reconciliation, promoting serenity and peace. They are the divine-human modes of healing of the sick, of presence and companion on the journey toward eternal life. Sacraments make holy the sacramental bond of intimate communion of life and love in marriage, and they confirm the sacred power of service to persons called to ordained ministry. Sacraments are in concordance with the nature of the human person and community, both needing signs and symbols to ritualize sacred meanings that cannot otherwise be experienced.

All sacraments are celebrations of life, through creative liturgies of culture, time and place, and are revealed in present sacred moments. They memorialize the connectedness of the universe in the creation of life and sustenance, affirming and renewing a harmony in life and living, and persons in community. They involve and are built on presence and, in the reflections of O'Donohue, of presence described as "creative and turbulent, a visible sign of invisible grace," existing nowhere else "in such intimate and frightening access to the mysterium" (1997, xvi). There are other forms of ritual such as blessings for the seasons, the crops, for planting and for harvesting, for the fishing fleets going out to sea. They are celebrated at special periods in the human life cycle, especially the onset of puberty and entry into adulthood. There isn't anything that cannot reveal the presence of the holy, despite the fact we are emerging from the modernism of Western culture where the dominant mechanistic metaphor prevailed over the sacred for centuries.

This work has been an attempt to go beyond a reductionist naturalism to see human persons, life and the whole universe in a context that acknowledges both the immanence and the transcendence of God. Within a sacred space, expanding with life and creativity, the human person is the universe become conscious of itself. The knowledge and wonderful technologies of science have enabled us to know ourselves and our place within this universe in ways never before available to us. Such knowledge is both a reminder of our incalculable dignity and of our awesome responsibility. Both are humbling.

The human person's truest name is *CARE*. Care, as the human mode of being, is a conceptualization of an ontology of caring, of who we are as persons in relationship with self, with God, with others and with the whole self-creating universe. Care is enacted and solemnized through relationships and the adventure of friendship, the latter described by O'Donohue as both creative and subversive force, "the sweet grace that liberates us to approach, recognize and inhabit this adventure" (xvii). O'Donohue reflects on the Celtic sense of ontological friendship, the Celtic imagination that articulates the inner friendship embracing nature, divinity, underworld and the human world as one. As he uses the word friendship, he notes its difference from what he calls the *tired* word *relationship* that, in popular form, can mean nothing more than me and my computer. Developing a phenomenology of friendship in a lyrical form, his work is a book of *Celtic wisdom*, reflected in its title, *Anam Cara*, a Gaelic term meaning *soul friend*. I trust that the sense in which relationship is used as reflective of the human mode of being in this work is not a tired word, but speaks to the inner longing and outer caring response of the human person and is captured in O'Donohue's inspirational language of friendship.

From the first edition of this book in 1987, the engagement has been an act of caring for me, and over time it evolved through a search for a clearer understanding of the meaning of human care. Initial reflections focused on the attributes of caring people, specifically on what caregivers do when they care. This was a fairly simple process but, while helpful, it did not adequately address the ontological question of the nature of caring in itself. A leap of insight came at the moment it was obvious that caring is the human mode of being. Personal experience and the experience of others, as well as events on the global scene, continue to challenge this insight that became the basic premise of this work.

In the daily course of events, caring is not immediately evident: it is often more obvious by its absence than by its presence in human affairs. Negative criticisms about the quality of care continue to question its viability within the health care system itself. While not a new phenomenon, experiences of discontent within and even disaffection with the health care system tend to be accented more at a time when caregivers in all fields are burdened by pressures not of their own making. It is hoped these are isolated events and have a legitimacy that can be recognized through action and appraisal. But the greatest threat of all comes from the impact of an indifference that stifles the desire and commitment of persons to care in situations over which they have no control. Does the workplace itself make it difficult, if not impossible to care? All is not well.

But, along with the reality of criticism and the concerns about poor quality of service in some health care facilities, everyday we experience evidence to the contrary. The commitment to excellence of doctors and nurses, and of other health professionals still prevails, despite the demands of time and crises, the shortage of staff and the unavailability of needed resources. As noted earlier in a publication edited by Phillips and Benner (1994), the authors, while conceding the crisis in health care, focus on the importance of affirming and restoring caring practices in the helping professions by highlighting the narratives that give them flesh. Caring does exist in health care—in many situations through the unrelenting determination of administrators, educators and practitioners. The care in health care can only be incarnated and preserved in the service of these persons. They too need to be cared for.

A new addition to this work, "Healing through Story," is intended to take our understanding of caring as the human mode of being beyond the boundaries of the health profession to image in new ways our place and responsibility within the universe. (*See* chapter 6.) We can grasp our identity as human beings in a manner never before enjoyed by humankind. But, in recent years, we have also become aware of the destructive force of human habitation on this planet over the past few centuries. We are latecomers, occupying this beautiful planet for only forty thousand of its fifteen-billion-year history. We are presently faced with the question: How long is it possible for life to continue on this earth? If we don't soon suspend activities already eliminating species, destroying land and polluting air and water at a speed that places at high risk all life systems, sustainability of the planet is in serious jeopardy. This is the imminent call of care, an ethical-moral responsibility of the highest order. Rosemary Radford Ruether, the author of books and articles about spirituality, women and ecology, makes a sobering observation:

> The time is short for major changes, if we are to save much of the biotic system of the earth that is in danger. The Worldwatch Institute estimates that we have about forty years for major global shifts to be carried out voluntarily (until 2030). After that time major disasters of famine and collapse of life systems, under the pressures of exploitative use, will take place, and there could well be very dangerous militaristic and totalitarian responses from threatened elites, as indeed is already happening (as cited in Vardey 1995, 677).

It is in the context of our contemporary world in crisis, in the face of personal, professional, national and global experiences, that the thesis of this work provides a ray of hope. To actualize this ray of hope, we have to move, challenge and, if need be, force ourselves to believe that caring is the human mode of being, that each human person, friend or enemy carries within the capacity to care. Each of us can do something. If we cannot change the whole health care system, we can transform the small unit in which we work. If we cannot reverse ecological damage on a global scale, we can do something as individuals and as professionals. We can respect and save water, control garbage and pollution, cooperate in recycling and composting programs, be advocates in the workplace for change in the environment, and support existing policies and initiate new ones. Once again, Rosemary Radford Ruether's words leave us with hope:

> Being rooted in love for our real communities of life and for our common mother, Gaia, can teach us patient passion, a passion that is not burnt out in season, but can be renewed season after season. Our revolution is not just for us, but for our children, for the generations of living beings to come. What we can do is to plant a seed, nurture a seed-bearing plant here and there, and hope for a harvest that goes beyond the limits of our powers and the span of our lives (Ibid., 678).

As caring persons, we examine the values by which we live, the values that motivate us, the values that drive our political, social and economic systems. As caring professionals we challenge the technological imperative that claims what can be done ought to be done, that tends to dehumanize rather than humanize. As persons whose identity is care, we reflect on whether the mores we subscribe to or fail to question are sufficient to ground or build the kind of community and world fit for our descendants. As caring educators, we strengthen the building blocks of professional education, so that it provides the foundation and the environment required to nurture and draw forth the capacity to care professionally. We know that the care in health care is embodied in virtuous acts and is both transforming and transformative, and that professional life and practice are molded by an ethic of relational responsibility. And all of us humanize our relationships through reflective practice, striving to become contemplatives in the midst of chaos.

Karl Rahner is often quoted as saying, "*We are always unfinished symphonies.*" This is a heartening statement for caring persons, whose sensitivity to the ever-increasing demands of ministry, find the challenges of every day often exceeding the energy and resources available to respond to them. But it is more profoundly a reminder about human life itself. We can only take on a small section of the vineyard at any one time, and this small corner may be all we are called to cultivate in our lifetime. This book itself is an unfinished symphony, the more so, as nearing its completion, there is so much more to say and so much already said that could have been said better. But it leads me to image the word symphony in another context—as apt metaphor for the universal call of care. Its development is for another time. A poem by Katie Eriksson provides a fitting conclusion.

> The well-springs of art are love, life, and suffering.
> Art emerges from the human spirit and mingles
> with the nuances of body and soul to form a work
> that mirrors the innermost being of a person, and
> the actual shaping of his/her existence.
>
> I want to create a symphony in major and minor keys
> with gladness, life, and suffering, sorrow and pain.
> Its name shall be Suffering.
>
> I want to form a work of art from the sparkling stars of heaven
> and the corals of the sea.
> Its name shall be Love.
>
> I want to paint a canvas that accommodates the goodness
> of the whole world and its beauty.
> Its name shall be Compassion.
>
> Speak to me about suffering, of your suffering.
> Speak so that it emerges in all its particularity
> with all of its nuances and ingredients.
> I will try to understand and within me form a figure
> of your suffering through my compassion.
>
> (Katie Eriksson, "Reflections on Suffering")

BIBLIOGRAPHY

Abbot, A. *The System of the Professions*. Chicago: University of Chicago Press, 1988. <http://www.advocateweb.org>

Aiken, H.D. *Reason and Conduct*. New York: Alfred A. Knopf, 1962.

Alexander, A. *The Antigonish Movement: Moses Coady and Adult Education Today*. Toronto: Thompson Educational Publishing, 1997.

Barber, B. "Some Problems in the Sociology of Professions." *Daedalus* 92 (1963): 672.

Baum, G. "Faith and Culture." *The Ecumenist* 24 (1985): 9-13.

Berry, T. "Christianity's Role in the Earth Project." In *Christianity and Ecology: Seeking the Well-being of Earth and Humans*, edited by D.T. Hessel and R. Radford Ruether, 127-134. Cambridge, MA: Harvard University Center for Study of World Religion, 2000; distributed by Harvard University Press.

_____. *Riverdale Papers*. Vol. 2, *The Ecological Age*. Riverdale, NY: Riverdale Center for Religious Research, 2000.

_____. *The Dream of the Earth*. San Francisco: Sierra Club Books, 1988.

_____. *Riverdale Papers*. Riverdale, NY: Riverdale Center for Religious Research, 1978.

Bok, S. *Lying: Moral Choice in Public and Private Life*. New York: Random House and Vintage Books, 1979.

Boykin, A. and S. Schoenhofer. "The Role of Nursing Leadership in Creating Caring Environments in Health Care Delivery Systems." *Administration Quarterly* 25 (2001): 1–7.

_____. *Nursing as Caring: A Model for Transforming Practice*. Boston: Jones and Bartlett, 2001.

Boykin, A. and M.E. Parker. "Illuminating Spirituality in the Classroom." In *Caring from the Heart: The Convergence of*

Caring and Spirituality, edited by M. Simone Roach, 21-33. New York/Mahwah, NJ: Paulist Press, 1997.

Brockett, M.M. "Building Trustworthy Relationships: A Reconstruction of Ethics Education for the Health Care Professions." PhD diss., Ontario Institute for Studies in Education, University of Toronto, 1997.

Bruteau, B. *God's Ecstacy: The Creation of a Self-creating World*. New York: Crossroad Publishing Company, 1997.

Cahill, L.S. *Sex, Gender, and Christian Ethics*. Cambridge, MA: Cambridge University Press, 1996.

———. "A 'Natural Law' Reconsideration of Euthanasia." *Linacre Quarterly* 44 (1977): 47-63.

Campbell, A.V. *Moderated Love: A Theology of Professional Care*. London: SPCK, 1984.

Canadian Conference of Catholic Bishops (CCCB). *Catechism of the Catholic Church*. Ottawa: Concacan, 1994.

Canadian Nurses Association. *Code of Ethics for Registered Nurses*. Ottawa: Canadian Nurses Association, 1997.

Canadian Oxford Dictionary. Edited by K. Barber. Toronto: Oxford University Press, 1999.

Capra, F. *The Turning Point: Science, Society and the Rising Culture*. Toronto: Bantam Books, 1982.

Carson, R. *Silent Spring*. New York: Houghton Mifflin Co.; Fawcett Crest Books, 1962.

Cassidy, S. *Sharing the Darkness: The Spirituality of Caring*. London: Darton, Longman and Todd, 1988.

Catholic Health Association of Canada (CHAC). *Health Ethics Guide*. Ottawa: Catholic Health Association of Canada, 2000.

Clarke, T. "The Divine in Our Present Revelatory Moment." In *Befriending the Earth: A Theology of Reconciliation between Humans and the Earth*, editd by S. Dunn and A. Lonergan, 29-37. Mystic, CT: Twenty-Third Publications, 1991.

Coady, M.M. *Masters of Their Own Destiny*. New York: Harper & Bros., 1939.

Conlon, J. *Earth Story: Sacred Story*. Mystic, CT: Twenty-Third Publications, 1994.

Donahue, M.P. *Nursing: The Finest Art: An Illustrated History*. Toronto: C.V. Mosby Company, 1985.

Dorr, D. *Integral Spirituality: Resources for Community, Justice, Peace and the Earth*. Maryknoll, NY: Orbis Books, 1990.

Dunn, S. and A. Lonergan, eds. *Befriending the Earth: A Theology of Reconciliation between Humans and the Earth*. Mystic, CT: Twenty-Third Publications, 1991.

Einstein, A. Circa. 1930s. <http://mcsc95.pld.com/projects98/kris/albert5.html>.

Eliot, T.S. *The Complete Poems and Plays, 1909-1950*. New York: Harcourt, Brace & World, 1971.

Eriksson, K. *Den Lidande Manniskan (The Suffering Human Being)*. Stockholm: Almqvist and Wiksell, 1994.

Fagothey, A. *Right and Reason: Ethics in Theory and Practice*. 6th ed. St. Louis, MO: C.V. Mosby Company, 1976.

Farley, M.S. *Personal Commitments: Beginning, Keeping, Changing*. New York: Harper & Row, 1986.

Feldstein, L.C. *Homo Querens: The Seeker and the Sought*. New York: Fordham University Press, 1978.

Fenton-Comack, M. "Ethical Issues in Critical Care: A Perceptual Study of Nurses' Attitudes, Beliefs and Ability to Cope." Master's thesis, University of Manitoba, Winnipeg, 1987.

Finley, J. *Merton's Palace of Nowhere: A Search for God through an Awareness of the True Self*. Notre Dame, IN: Ave Maria Press, 1978.

Fox, M. *A Spirituality Named Compassion*. Minneapolis, MN: Winston Press, 1979.

Frankl, V.E. *Man's Search for Meaning*. New York: Pocket Books, 1959.

Franklin, U.M. *The Real World of Technology*. rev. ed. CBC Massey Lecture Series. Toronto: CBC Enterprises, 1990.

Freidson, E. "Professionalism, Caring, and Nursing." Paper prepared for Park Lodge Center, Park Ridge, Illinois, 1990. <http://itsa.ucsf.edu/~eliotf/professionalism,_caring,_a.html> (26 September 2001).

_____. *The Profession of Medicine*. Chicago: University of Chicago Press, 1988.

_____. *Professional Powers: A Study of the Institutionalization of Formal Knowledge*. Chicago: University of Chicago Press, 1986.

Freshwater, D. "Communicating with Self through Caring: The Student Nurse's Experience of Reflective Practice." *International Journal for Human Caring* 3 (1999): 28-33.

Garesché, E.F. *Ethics and the Art of Conduct for Nurses*. Philadelphia: W.B. Saunders, 1929.

Gateley, E. *Psalms of a Laywoman*. Trabuco Canyon, CA: Source Books, 1981.

Gaut, D.A. *Historical Review of the IAHC 1978-1993*. Paoli, PA: International Association for Human Caring, 1993.

Gaylin, W. *Caring*. New York, Alfred A. Knopf, 1979.

Gonsiorek, J., ed. *The Breach of Trust: Sexual Exploitation by Health Care Professionals and Clergy*. Thousand Oaks, CA: Sage Publishing, 1995.

Gula, R.M. *The Good Life: Where Morality and Spirituality Converge*. New York/Mahwah, NJ: Paulist Press, 1999.

_____. *Ethics in Pastoral Ministry*. New York/Mahwah, NJ: Paulist Press, 1996.

_____. *Reason Informed by Faith: Foundations of Catholic Morality*. New York/Mahwah, NJ: Paulist Press, 1989.

Gustafson, J. *Ethics from a Theocentric Perspective.* Chicago: University of Chicago Press, 1982.

Haring, B. *Free and Faithful in Christ: Moral Theology for Clergy and Laity.* Vol. 1. New York: Seabury Press; A Crossroad Book, 1978.

Hauerwas, S. "On Medicine and Virtue: A Response." In *Virtue and Medicine: Explorations in the Character of Medicine*, edited by E.E. Shelp, 347-355. Boston: D. Reidel Publishing Co., 1985.

_____. *A Community of Character: Toward a Constructive Christian Social Ethic.* Notre Dame, IN: University of Notre Dame Press, 1981.

Heidegger, M. *Being and Time.* Translated by J. Macquarrie and E. Robinson. London: SCM Press, 1962.

Hellegers, A. "Compassion and Competence." *America* 133 (1975): 113.

Heschel, A.J. *Who Is Man?* Stanford, CA: Stanford University Press, 1965.

Hessel, D.T. and R. Radford Ruether, eds. *Christianity and Ecology: Seeking the Well-being of Earth and Humans.* Cambridge, MA: Harvard Center for Study of World Religions, distributed by Harvard University Press, 2000.

Hiebert, T. "The Human Vocation: Origins and Transformations in Christian Traditions." In *Christianity and Ecology: Seeking the Well-being of Earth and Humans*, edited by D.T. Hessel and R. Radford Ruether, 134-154. Cambridge, MA: Harvard Center for Study of World Religions, distributed by Harvard University Press, 2000.

Holland, J. "The Post-Modern Paradigm Implicit in the Church's Shift to the Left." In *The Faith That Transforms*, edited by M.J. Leddy, 39-61. New York: Paulist Press, 1987.

Irons, R. "The Sexually Exploitive Professional: An Addiction Sensitive Model for Assessment." Monograph presented at the Second Annual Conference on Addiction: Prevention,

Recognition, Treatment, to the Behaviorial Care Network and Abbot Northwestern Hospital, Minneapolis, Minnesota, November 1991.

Irons, R. and J.P. Schneider. *The Wounded Healer: Addiction-Sensitive Approach to theSexually Exploitive Professional*. N.P.: Jason Aronson Publishers, 1999.

Jersild, A.T. *The Psychology of Adolescence*. New York: Macmillan Publishing Company, 1957.

Jonas, H. *Philosophical Essays: From Ancient Creed to Technological Man*. Chicago: University of Chicago Press; Midway Reprint, 1974.

Johns, C. "Catlin's Story: Realizing Caring within Everyday Practice through Guided Reflections." *International Journal for Human Caring* 1(1997): 33-39.

Johns, C. and D. Freshwater, eds. *Transforming Nursing through Reflective Practice*. Oxford, England: Blackwell Science, 1998.

Johnson, E.A. "Losing and Finding Creation in the Christian Tradition." In *Christianity and Ecology: Seeking the Well-being of Earth and Humans*, edited by D.T. Hessel and R. Radford Ruether, 3-21. Cambridge, MA: Harvard Center for Study of World Religions, distributed by Harvard University Press, 2000.

Kaiser, S.B. *The Social Psychology of Clothing: Symbolic Appearances in Context*. 2d ed. New York: Macmillan Publishing Company, 1985.

Keenan, J.F. "Virtue Ethics." In *Christian Ethics: An Introduction*, edited by B. Hoose, 84-94. Collegeville, MN: Liturgical Press, 1998.

Kelsey, M. *Caring*. New York: Paulist Press, 1981.

Kownacki, M. L. *The Blue Heron and Thirty-Seven Other Miracles*. Erie, PA: Benetvision Press, 1996.

Krathwohl, D.R., B.S. Bloom and B.M. Bertam. *Taxonomy of*

Educational Objectives: Affective Domain. 2 vols. New York: David McKay, 1964.

Kultgen, J. *Ethics and Professionalism.* Philadelphia: University of Pennsylvania Press, 1988.

Laidlaw, A.F. *The Campus and the Community.* Montreal: Harvest House, 1961.

Lakeland, P. *Postmodernity.* Minneapolis, MN: Fortress Press, 1997.

Le Fanu, J. "Blinded by Science." *The Tablet* (2 Dec 2000): 1628-1629. <http://www.the tablet.co.uk/cgi-bin/archive_db.cgi?tablet-00500>.

Leininger, M. M. *Transcultural Nursing: Concepts, Theories, Research, and Practices.* 2d ed. New York: McGraw-Hill Custom College Series, 1995.

_____. "Humanism, Health and Cultural Values." In *Health Care Issues,* edited by Madeleine M. Leininger, 37-60. Philadelphia: F.A. Davis, 1974.

_____. *Nursing and Anthropology: Two Worlds to Blend.* New York: John Wiley and Sons, 1970.

Leininger, M. and C.L. Reynolds. *Cultural Care Diversity and Universality.* New York: Urban & Fischer, 2000.

Lerman, H. "Preface." In *Breach of Trust: Sexual Exploitation by Health Care Professionals and Clergy,* edited by J. Gonsiorek, ix-xi. Thousand Oaks, CA: Sage Publishing, 1995.

Loftus, J.A. *Understanding Sexual Misconduct by Clergy: A Handbook for Ministers.* Washington, D.C.: Pastoral Press, 1994.

Lonergan, A. and C. Richards, eds. *Thomas Berry and the New Cosmology.* Mystic, CT: Twenty-Third Publications, 1987.

Lonergan, B. *Method in Theology.* London: Darton, Longman & Todd, 1971. Reprint. Toronto: University of Toronto for Lonergan Research Institute of Regis College, 1990.

Lotz, J. and M. Welton. *Father Jimmy: Life and Times of Jimmy Tompkins*. Sydney, NS: Breton Books, 1997.

MacDonald, K. *The Sociology of the Professions*. London: Sage Publishing, 1995.

MacIntyre, A. *After Virtue: A Study in Moral Theory*. Notre Dame, IN: University of Notre Dame Press, 1981.

Maguire, D.C. "Population, Consumption, Ecology: The Triple Problematic." In *Christianity and Ecology: Seeking the Wellbeing of Earth and Humans*, edited by D.T. Hessel and R. Radford Ruether, 403-427. Cambridge, MA: Harvard Center for Study of World Religions, distributed by Harvard University Press, 2000.

_____. *The Moral Choice*. New York: Doubleday & Company, 1978.

Malin, N., ed. *Professionalism, Boundaries and the Workplace*. New York: Routledge, 2000.

May, R. *Love and Will*. New York: W.W. Norton & Co., 1969.

_____. *Man's Search for Himself*. New York: W.W. Norton & Co., 1953.

Mayeroff, M. *On Caring*. New York: Harper & Row, 1971; New York: Perennial Library, 1972.

McLaughlin, D. "Silent Spring Revisited." *PBS Online and WGBH/Frontline*.1998.<http://www.pbs.org/wgbh/pages/frontline/shows/nature/disrupt/sspring.html> (26 September 2001).

Milgrom, J.H. *Boundaries in Professional Relationships*. Minneapolis, MN: Walk-in Counseling Center, 1992.

Miller, J.P. *The Contemplative Practitioner: Meditation in Education for the Professions*. Toronto: OISE Press, 1994.

Mische, P. "Toward a Global Spirituality." *Whole Earth Papers* 16 (1982): 4–15.

Moltmann, J. *God in Creation: A New Theology of Creation and the Spirit of God*. 1st U.S. ed. Translated by Margaret Kohl. San Francisco: Harper & Row, Publishers, 1985.

New American Bible. Translated by members of the Catholic Biblical Association of America. New York: Thomas Nelson Inc., 1971.

Niebuhr, H.R. *The Responsible Self: An Essay in Christian Moral Philosophy.* New York: Harper & Row Publishers, 1978.

Nolan, A. *Jesus before Christianity.* London: Darton, Longman, and Todd; Maryknoll, NY: Orbis Books, 1978.

Nouwen, H.J.M. *Life of the Beloved: Spiritual Living in a Secular World.* New York: Crossroad Publishing Company, 1992.

_____. "Compassion." Unpublished manuscript, Yale University, New Haven, Connecticut, 1980.

_____. *The Wounded Healer.* New York: Doubleday & Co., Image Books, 1979.

_____. *Out of Solitude.* Notre Dame, IN: Ave Maria Press, 1974.

Nouwen, H.J.M., D.P. McNeill and D.A. Morrison. *Compassion: A Reflection on the Christian Life.* 1st ed. Garden City, NY: Doubleday, 1982; Image Books, 1983.

O'Brien, M.E. *Spirituality in Nursing: Standing on Holy Ground.* Boston: Jones and Bartlett Publishers, 1999.

O'Connell, T.E. *Making Disciples: A Handbook of Christian Moral Formation.* New York: Crossroad Publishing Company, 1998.

_____. *Principles for a Catholic Morality.* New York: Seabury Press, A Crossword Book, 1976.

O'Donohue, J. *Anam Cara: A Book of Celtic Wisdom.* New York: HarperCollins, Publishers, 1997.

O'Sullivan, E. *Transformative Learning: Educational Vision for the 21st Century.* Toronto: University of Toronto Press, 1999.

Parker, M.E. and C. Barry. "Community Practice Guided by a Nursing Model." *Nursing Science Quarterly* 12 (1999): 125-131.

Patrick, A.E. *Liberating Conscience: Feminist Explorations in Catholic Moral Theology.* New York: Continuum Publishing Company, 1996.

Pellegrino, E.D. "The Virtuous Physician, and the Ethics of Medicine." In *Virtue and Medicine: Explorations in the Character of Medicine*, edited by E.E. Shelp, 237-255. Boston: D. Reidel Publishing Co., 1985.

Pellegrino, E.D. and D.C. Thomasma. *The Christian Virtues in Medical Practice*. Washington, D.C.: Georgetown University Press, 1996.

Pellegrino, E.D., R.M. Veatch and J.P. Langan, eds. *Ethics, Trust, and the Professions: Philosophical and Cultural Aspects*. Washington, D.C.: Georgetown University Press, 1991.

Pharr, S.J. and R.D. Putnam, eds. *Disaffected Democracies: What's Troubling the Trilateral Democracies?* Princeton, NJ: Princeton University Press, 2000.

Phillips, S.S. and P. Benner. *The Crisis of Care: Affirming and Restoring Caring Practices in the Helping Professions*. Washington, D.C.: Georgetown University Press, 1994.

Post, S.G. *Spheres of Love: Toward a New Ethics of the Family*. Dallas: Southern Methodist University Press, 1994.

_____. *A Theory of Agape: On the Meaning of Christian Love*. Toronto: Associated University Presses, 1990.

Radford Ruether, R. "Ecofeminism: The Challenge to Theology." In *Christianity and Ecology: Seeking the Well-being of Earth and Humans*, edited by D.T. Hessel and R. Radford Ruether, 96-112. Cambridge, MA: Harvard Center for Study of World Religions, distributed by Harvard University Press, 2000.

_____. "Gaia and God." In *God in All Worlds: An Anthology of Contemporary Spiritual Writing*, edited by L. Vardey, 678. New York: Random House, Inc.; Vintage Books, 1995.

_____. *Gaia and God*. New York: HarperCollins Publishers, 1992.

Ramsey, P. *The Patient as Person*. New Haven, CT: Yale University Press, 1970.

Random House College Dictionary. rev. ed. Edited by J. Stein. New York: Random House, 1965.

Roach, M. Simone, ed. *Caring from the Heart: The Convergence of Caring and Spirituality.* New York/Mahwah, NJ: Paulist Press, 1997.

———. "Caring: The Human Mode of Being: Implications for Nursing." In *Perspectives on Caring: Monograph 1.* Toronto: University of Toronto Faculty of Nursing, 1984.

———. "Reflections on a Code of Ethics for Nurses in Canada." Paper prepared for the Canadian Nurses Association, Ottawa, 1981.

———. "Toward a Value Oriented Curriculum with Implications for Nursing Education." PhD diss., Catholic University of America, Washington, D.C., 1970.

Rolheiser, R. *The Holy Longing: The Search for a Christian Spirituality.* New York: Doubleday, 1999.

Rowe, S.C. *Living beyond Crisis: Essays on Discovery and Being in the World.* New York: Pilgrim Press, 1980.

Russell, P. *The White Hole in Time.* New York: HarperCollins Publishers, 1992.

Scharper, S.B. *Redeeming the Time: A Political Theory of the Environment.* New York: Continuum Publishers, 1997.

Scharper, S.B. and H. Cunningham, eds. *The Green Bible.* Maryknoll, NY: Orbis Books, 1993.

Schmitt, R. *Martin Heidegger on Being Human.* New York: Random Books, 1969.

Schneiders, S.M. "Spirituality, Religion and Theology: Mapping the Terrain, Part 1." Presented at the Sisters, Servants of the Immaculate Heart of Mary (IHM) Theological Education Project, Cycle 3, Monroe, MI, summer 1999. <http://www.ihmsisters.org/ spirituality-theological.html> (21 September 2001).

Schoener, G.R. "Historical Overview." In *Breach of Trust: Sexual Exploitation by Health Care Professionals and Clergy*, edited by J.C. Gonsiorek, 3-17. Thousand Oaks, CA: Sage Publishing, 1995.

Schon, Donald A. *Educating the Reflective Practitioner: Toward a New Design for Teaching and Learning in the Professions.* 1st ed. San Francisco: Jossey-Bass Publishers, 1987.

_____. *The Reflective Practitioner: How Professionals Think in Action.* New York: Basic Books, 1983.

Selling, J. "The Human Person." In *Christian Ethics: An Introduction,* edited by B. Hoose, 97-109. Collegeville, MN: Liturgical Press, 1998.

Shelp, E.E., ed. *Virtue and Medicine: Explorations in the Character of Medicine.* Boston: C. Reidel Publishing Co., 1985.

Shils, E. "The Sanctity of Life." *Encounter* 26 (1967): 39-49.

Smith, H. *Beyond the Post-Modern Mind.* New York: Crossroad Publishing Company, 1982.

Solzhenitsyn, A.I. *The Gulag Archipelago.* New York: Westview Press, 1997.

_____. *A World Split Apart.* New York: Harper & Row, Publishers, 1978.

Somerville, Margaret. *The Ethical Canary: Science, Society and the Human Spirit.* Toronto: Penguin Books, 2000.

Sorokin, P. *The Crisis of Our Age.* New York: E.P. Dutton, 1942.

Spohn, W.C. *Go and Do Likewise: Jesus and Ethics.* New York: Continuum Publishing Company, 1999.

Swimme, B. *The Universe a Green Dragon: A Cosmic Creation Story.* Sante Fe: NM, Bear & Company, 1988.

Swimme, B. and T. Berry. "The Universe Story: A New, Celebratory Cosmology." *Amices Journal* (Winter 1993): 30-31.

_____. *The Universe Story: From Primordial Flaring Forth to the Ecozoic Era: A Celebration of the Unfolding of the Cosmos.* New York: HarperCollins, Publisher, 1992.

Tarnas, R. *The Passion of the Western Mind: Understanding the Ideas*

That Have Shaped Our World. New York: Ballantine Books, 1991.

Teilhard de Chardin, P. *The Divine Milieu: An Essay on the Interior Life.* New York: Harper and Row, 1960.

──── . *The Phenomenon of Man.* London: W. Collins & Sons Co., 1959.

Tillard, J.M.R. "The Health World: A Place for the Following of Christ." *Lumen Vitae: International Review of Religious Education* 36 (1981): 7-44.

Toulmin, S. *Cosmopolis: The Hidden Agenda of Modernity.* New York: Free Press, 1990.

Tournier, P. *The Meaning of Persons.* Translated by E. Hudson. New York: Harper & Row, 1957.

von Hildebrand, D. *Christian Ethics.* New York: David McKay Co., 1953a.

──── . *The New Tower of Babel.* New York: P.J. Kennedy & Sons, 1953b.

Wagner, A. Lynn. "Connecting to Nurse-Self through Reflective Poetic Story." *International Journal for Human Caring* 4 (2000): 7-12.

──── . "Within the Circle of Death: Transpersonal Poetic Reflections on Nurses' Stories about the Quality of the Dying Process." *International Journal for Human Caring* 3 (1999): 21-30.

Watson, J. *Postmodern Nursing and Beyond.* New York: Harcourt Brace and Co., 1999.

Wilbur, K. *A Brief History of Everything.* Boston: Shambhala Publications, 1996.

Winter, G. *Liberating Creation: Foundations of Religious Social Ethics.* New York: Crossroad Publishing Company, 1981.

Wright, R.A. *Human Values in Health Care: The Practice of Ethics.* Toronto: McGraw-Hill Book Company, 1987.

Wuthnow, R. *Act of Compassion: Caring for Others and Helping Ourselves*. Princeton, NJ: Princeton University Press, 1991.

Zaner, R.M. "The Phenomenon of Trust and the Patient-Physician Relationship." In *Ethics, Trust, and the Professions: Philosophical and Cultural Aspects*, edited by E.D. Pellegrino, R.M. Veatch and J.P. Langan, 45-67. Washington, D.C.: Georgetown University Press, 1991.

VIDEOTAPES

Canticle to the Cosmos with Brian Swimme [video]. 12 videotapes. Produced by Newstory Project and distributed by Tides Foundation, Livermore, California, 1990.

The Global Brain [video]. Produced by P. Russell and Chris Hall Productions. Distributed by Penny Price Media, Staatsbury, NY, n.d.

The Greening of Faith: Ethics [video]. Program 2. Produced and distributed by Cathedral Films and Video, Westlake Village, CA, 1993.

The Greening of Faith: Theology and Spirituality [video]. Program 1. Produced and distributed by Cathedral Films and Video, Westlake Village, CA, 1993.

The Hidden Heart of the Cosmos [video]. Produced by B. Swimme. Distributed by Center for the Story of the Universe, Mill Valley, CA, 1996.

Spirit and Nature [television program]. Interview with S. McFague by Bill Moyers. Produced and directed by Gail Pellett. Aired on Public Broadcasting System.

The Unfolding Story [video]. Narrated by Mike Farrell. Produced by Raylands Production. Distributed by Foundation for Global Community, Paolo Alto, CA, 1993.

INDEX

A

Affective domain
 in commitment, 62
Affective response. *See also* Affectivity
 and "being affected," 128–130
 and moral conscience, 60–61
Affectivity. *See also* Affective response;
  D. von Hildebrand
 nature of, 129
 spiritual power of, 129
Agape
 reflections on. *See* S. Post
 understanding of, 11
Anam Cara (J. O'Donohue, 1987), 140
The Antigonish Movement
 and Moses Coady, 26
Anthropocentrism, 105
Anthropological questions on caring, 42
Attributes of caring. *See* Caring
Autonomy
 personal, 136
 as a right to self-determination, 71

B

Being-in-the-world, 30, 55
Benner, Patricia, 95, 134–135. *See also*
  The Crisis of Care
Berry, Thomas
 and the future of the universe, 106
 and the universe story, 103–107
*The Blue Heron and Thirty-Seven Other
  Miracles* (M. Kownacki, 1996), 1
Bok, Sissela
 and the decline in public confidence, 56
Breach of Trust (J. Gonsiorek, 1995), 88
Boykin, Anne, 125

C

Cahill, Lisa
 and gender, 12
The call of care, 93–97
Canadian Catholic Organization for
  Development and Peace, 23
Canadian Conference of Catholic
  Bishops, 23, 24
Canadian Nurses Association

*Codes of Ethics for Registered
  Nurses*, 57–58, 71–72
Care
 opportunities to, 35
 the Roman myth of, 38
 of the sick. *See* Christians
Caregiver
 and caring for self, 34, 132
Caregivers. *See* Nursing
Caring. *See also The Crisis of Care;*
  Nursing; Person/individual;
  Reflections on Caring
 attributes of, 39, 43–49, 50–66. *See
  also* The SIX Cs
 and community, 23–25
 a conceptualization of, 38–40
 and dependency, 127, 128
 as grounded in religio. *See* Religio
 and the "helping" professions, 30. *See
  also* Professions and
  professionalism
 as the human mode of being, 3, 7,
  23–27, 28, 42
 the limitations of, 62–63
 as love, 7. *See also* Love
 ontology of, 41–43
 professional, 11
 in professional education. *See*
  Transformative learning
 and professional ethics, 67–68
 the professionalization of, 39
 and the professions, 39–40
 reflections on. *See* Reflections
 as response to dependency. *See* W.
  Gaylin
 as response to value, 125–126. *See
  also* D. von Hildebrand
 the SIX Cs of. *See* SIX Cs
 the universe of. *See* The universe
 as virtuous activity, 4
Caring behaviors, 43. *See also* Caring
  events; Professional caring
Caring events. *See also* Disasters
 and the community response to,
  23–25, 26
 and the personal impact of, 23–24

159

INDEX

Caring ontology, 41–42, 42–43
Caring people, 25, 26
Caring and professional ethics, 67–81.
　See also Ethical discernment;
　Ethics; Virtue ethics
　and the case study, 79–80
　the language of, 69–70
　noblesse oblige in, 67, 68, 73, 77
Caring professions. See Professions
　and professionalism
Caring universe, 41–43. See also The
　universe
Cartesian dualism, 121
Case study
　and the attributes of caring, 43–49
　and the process used, 45
　questions about, 49
　and reflections on professional
　　ethics, 79–80
　responses to, 45–48
　at St. Martha's Regional Hospital, 43,
　　49
　and the SIX Cs. See SIX Cs
　and spiritual care, 49
Chaos
　as change, 1
Christ. See Jesus Christ
Christ rooms, 121
Christianity and ecology, 107
Christians
　and care of the sick, 120–121
Codes of ethics
　for nursing. See Canadian Nurses
　　Association
　for research, 56–57
　violation of, 57
Commitment
　and caring, 62–64
　and the case study, 48
　definition of, 62
　and devotion. See M. Mayeroff
　and learning, 131–132
Compassion. See also R. Gula; H.
　　Nouwen
　as an attribute of caring, 26, 39, 53
　and the case study, 45–46
　for the Christian, 51
　definition of, 50
　of the earth. See J. Conlon

　and humam sexuality. See M. Fox
　and Jesus Christ, 51
　and learning, 131–132
　in public life, 50–51
　as a relationship, 51
　versus competitiveness, 51
　in volunteerism, 26
Competence. See also Nursing
　and caring, 54, 55
　and the case study, 46
　definition of, 54
　and learning, 131–132
　threat to, 54–55
Comportment. See also S. Kaiser
　and caring, 64–66
　and the case study, 48
　dress and language in, 64
　and learning, 131–132
Confidence
　and caring, 56–58
　and the case study, 46–47
　decline in. See S. Bok
　definition of, 56
　and learning, 131–132
　and the professions, 86, 87
　and the use of deception, 58
Confidentiality
　as an ethical problem, 79
Conlon, James
　on compassion of the earth, 53
Conscience. See also R. Gula
　and caring, 58–61
　and the case study, 47
　collective, 58–59
　definition of, 60
　description of, 60
　in the Freudian school, 59
　individual, 12–13, 58
　and learning, 131–132
　in professional caring, 60
"Cosmic Walk," 111–115
Contemplation. See Practice
Covenant
　and contract relationships, 75–76
The Creation Story. See also The
　　Universe Story
　as gratuitous love, 7–8
　in Judaism-Christianity, 7
　and the new story, 8, 14, 109–111

The Crisis of Care (S. Phillips and P. Benner, 1994), 12
Cure/care dichotomy, 30
Customs
　as etiquette, 69
　ethical, 69

D
de Chardin, Teilhard
　the thinking of, 102
　and the universe, 14
Devotion, 29
Disasters. *See also* Caring events
　in Nicaragua, 25, 26
　at Peggy's Cove, 24, 25–26, 27
Dooley, Tom, 25
Dorr, Donal
　on spirituality, 9–10
Dress and language
　as symbols of communication, 64, 65
Duplicity
　in health care, 57, 58
　in public life, 56

E
Ecozoic era, 103
Educating the Reflective Practitioner (D. Schon, 1987), 133
Education and practice. *See also* Affective response and "being affected"; Practice; Transformative learning
　holistic, 135–136
　for professional caring, 117–137
　and the reform of, 123
　as transformative, 117–120
Einstein, Albert
　on technological development, 19
　and the transformation of science, 110
Eisley, Loren, 61
Elliot Allen Institute for Theology and Ecology (Toronto), 14
Engineering. *See also* H. Jonas
　biological, 17
　definition of, 17
　genetic, 17
　human, 17
　mechanical, 17

Epistemological questions on caring, 42
Epistemology, 42
Eriksson, Katie. *See* "Reflections on Suffering"
Ethical discernment. *See also* Caring and professional ethics; Ethics; Virtue ethics
　in health care practice, 78
　models for, 77–79
Ethics. *See also* Caring and professional ethics; Ethical discernment, Virtue ethics
　in contemporary discussion, 70–71
　and customs, 69
　as a discipline of knowledge, 70–73
　in education, 118–119
　and moral behavior, 69–70
　and the moral life, 70-80
　origin of, 69
　as a process of discernment, 77–80
　and relational responsibility, 73–76
　theories of. *See* H.R. Niebuhr
Ethics and the Art of Conduct for Nurses (E.F. Garesché, 1929), 67
Ethics and morals, 69–70

F
Farley, M.
　forms of commitment, 63–64
Franklin, Dr. Ursula
　and understanding technology, 15–16
Florida Atlantic University, 125
Fox, Matthew
　on compassion and human sexuality, 52–53
　on competence, 54–55
Frankl, Viktor
　and dehumanization, 37. *See Man's Search for Meaning*
Freidson, Eliot
　and modes of work, 91–93, 96–97
Freshwater, Dawn
　and reflective practice, 133

G
Gandhi, Mahatma, 25
Garesché, Edward F.
　on ethics for nurses, 67

INDEX

Gaylin, Willard
  and the development of caring in humans, 30–32
  on caring and dependency, 126, 128
Gately, Edwina
  and "The Sharing," 99–101
God
  the compassion of, 51
Gonsiorek, John C.
  and breach of trust in professions, 58
  physician-patient sex, 89
Gula, R.M.
  on compassion and care of self, 53
  on conscience, 59–60
The Gulag Archipelago (A. Solzhenitsyn), 36, 37

H

Healing through story, 99–115. *See also* "Cosmic Walk"
Health care
  and the Christian tradition, 120, 121
  the goals of, 136
  and the Hebrew tradition, 120
  in a historical context, 120–122
  a model for, 10
  as a moral enterprise, 2, 68
  as a personal-communal service, 120
  and technology. *See* Technology
Health care professions. *See* Professions and professionalism
Health care system
  barriers in, 68
  crisis in, 94, 141–142
  evidence of caring in, 95, 142
  quality of care in, 4, 141
  state of, 4
  workplace. *See* Workplace structures
Helping professions. *See* Professions and professionalism
Higgins, Michael
  on human cloning, 18
  and use of technology, 19
The Holy Longing (R. Rolheiser, 1999)
  and the person, 8
Human cloning. *See also* Michael Higgins; Dr. Margaret Somerville
  challenges to, 18–19
  ethics of, 18–19
  motives for, 16–17
Human suffering, 14–15
  as evil, 15
  relief of, 15
Humphrey, Hubert, 50-51

I

Important-in-itself
  as response to value, 129
Individualism
  versus altruism, 26
International Association for Human Caring, 134–135
International Journal for Human Caring, 134

J

Jesus. *See* Jesus Christ
Jesus Christ
  and care of the sick, 121
  and the miracles of, 51
Jonas, Hans
  reflections on technological development, 17–18
Johns, Christopher
  and reflective practice, 133–134

K

Kaiser, S.
  studies in appearance, 65–66
Kownacki, Mary Lou
  The Blue Heron and Thirty-Seven Other Miracles, 1
  "Poem One," 1
  and sacrament, 139

L

Leininger, Madeleine, Dr.
  and cultural care diversity, 10
  and the first caring conference, 134
Lonergan, Bernard
  and the transcendental method, 21
Love. *See also* Agape; The Creation Story
  and the desire for, 10-11
  as human caring, 7
  madly in love, 8–9
  perversions of, 12
  and professional care, 22

and sexuality, 12
in special relations, 11
and spirituality. *See* Spirituality

M
MacIntyre, A.
  and the critique of Western philosophy, 73
Maguire, Daniel C.
  and the moral experience, 60
  and the threats to earth, 107–108
Making Disciples: A Handbook of Christian Moral Formation (T. O'Connell, 1998), 117
Mance, Jeanne, 25
Man's Search for Meaning (V. Frankl, 1959), 36
Marxism, 121
May, Rollo, 32
  and the inability to care, 33
Mayeroff, Milton
  on caring, 29, 97–98. *See also On Caring*
  on the quality of devotion, 62–63
Merton, Thomas
  and spirituality, 9
Moral theology
  teaching of. *See* T. O'Connell
Mother Theresa, 25

N
Natural law
  Catholic tradition of, 73–74
New Testament
  miracles of Jesus, 51
The New Tower of Babel (D. von Hildebrand, 1953), 129
Niebuhr, H. Richard
  and the critique of deontological and teleological theories, 74
Nouwen, Henri J.M.
  and compassion, 35, 50, 51–52
Nursing
  and caring, 95–96
  competence in, 54
  as the professionalization of caring, 67
  and reflective practice, 133, 134, 136.
    See also D. Freshwater
  training, 136

Nursing Reflection Conference, June 1998, 99

O
O'Brien, Mary Elizabeth
  Spirituality in Nursing: Standing on Holy Ground, 5–6
O'Connell, Timothy. *See also Making Disciples*
  and caring as value itself, 129–130
  and moral theology, 117
O'Donohue, J. *See also Anam Cara*
  and the Celtic imagination, 140–141
  and the sacraments, 139
On Caring (M Mayeroff, 1971), 97
Ontical expression of caring, 131–132.
  See also Six Cs
Ontical questions on caring, 42, 66
Onticological questions on caring, 41-42
Onticology, 42
Ontology, 42-43, 83

P
The Patient as Person (P. Ramsay, 1970), 76
Paul. *See* St. Paul
Pedagogical questions on caring, 42
Person/individual. *See also* Conscience; *The Holy Longing;* Human suffering; Paul Tournier; Technology
  and love. *See* Love
  in relation to others, 12-13
  as sacred, 8
  and technology, 15–21
  from the thoughts of St. Irenaeus (circa 165–200), 8
Phillips, Susan, 95. *See also* Caring, *The Crisis of Care*
Picard, Dr. Carol
  and the "Cosmic Walk." *See* "Cosmic Walk"
Pluralism
  in Western society, 121
Postmodern Nursing and Beyond (J. Watson, 1999), 123-124
Post, Stephen
  and reflections on agape, 11

163

Power. *See* Professions and professionalism
Practice of hospitality, 120
Practice. *See also* Education and practice; D. Schon; Transformative learning
  contemplative/reflective, 133–137
  the experience of reflective, 133
Professional caring
  and education. *See* Education and practice
  as moderated love, 22
Professional malpractice. *See also* Trust and boundary violations
  and confidence, 87
  visibility of, 85, 89
Professionalism, Caring and Nursing (E. Freidson, 1990), 91
Professions and professionalism. *See also* Trust and boundary violations
  and authentic respect, 87
  classical, 83, 87
  codes of ethics for, 85, 86. *See also* Canadian Nurses Association
  fiduciary relationship of, 85–86
  licensure of, 85
  noblesse oblige in, 84. *See also* Caring and professional ethics
  power and control in, 86, 88, 90
  rehabilitation for, 88–89
  sexual misconduct in. *See* Trust and boundary violations
  trust in, 84–85, 86–87. *See also* Trust and boundary violations
Public confidence
  decline in, 56

R
Radford Ruether, Rosemary
  and ecofeminism, 109, 142, 143
Rahner, Karl, 143–144
Ramsey, Paul, 76
Reflections on caring
  approach to, 21–22
"Reflections on Suffering," (K. Eriksson, 1994), 144
The Reflective Practitioner (D. Schon, 1983), 133

Religio. *See also* D. von Hildebrand
  and caring, 3
  and science and technology, 19
Research
  on caring, 34–35
Respect
  in caring for the body, 2–3
  for human dignity, 3
Rolheiser, Ronald
  and spirituality, 9
Roman myth. *See* Care

S
St. Paul, 70
Sacraments. *See also* J. O'Donahue
  as celebrations of life, 139–140
  description of, 2
  in faith traditions, 2
  of healing, 2
  as ritual of, 140
  of the Roman Catholic Church, 139
Sacredness
  of the individual, 8
Scharper, S.B.
  and the global crisis, 108
Schneiders, Sandra
  on spirituality, 9
Schon, Donald A.
  and reflective practice, 133
Self-determination
  a person's right to, 2
Sisters of St. Martha of Antigonish, 24
SIX Cs. *See also* Commitment; Compassion; Competence; Comportment; Confidence; Conscience; Transformative learning
  in the case study, 44–48
  evolution of, 43–44
  further elaboration of, 50–66
  the practice of. *See* Transformative learning
Solzhenitsyn, Aleksandr, 36–37
Somerville, Dr. Margaret
  on human cloning, 18–19
Spirituality. *See also* Donal Dorr; Thomas Merton; Ronald Rolheiser; Sandra Schneiders
  in Christianity, 9

definition of. *See* Sandra Schneiders
of the earth. *See* J. Conlon
in nursing. *See Spirituality in Nursing*
in other faiths, 9–10
from the prophet Micah, 10
Spirituality in Nursing: Standing on Holy Ground (M.E. O'Brien, 1999), 5–6
Supremacy of reason, 106, 121
Sustainability
of the planet, 102–103, 123
Sweitzer, Albert, 25
Swimme, Brian
and the universe story, 103, 104

T

Technology. *See also* Person/individual
current use of, 16-19
developments in, 16–19
and health care, 16–19
and religio. *See* Religio
and the technological imperative, 16
understanding of. *See* Dr. Ursula Franklin
and the universe, 21
Transformative learning. *See also* Affective response and "being affected"; Education and practice
and caring as response to value, 124–128
and caring as virtuous action, 130
the global perspective, 122–124
and the practice of the SIX Cs, 131–132
reflective and contemplative practice of, 133–137
Transformative Learning Centre, University of Toronto, 122–123
Transformative Learning: Educational Vision for the 21st Century (E. O'Sullivan, 1999), 123
Transforming Nursing through Reflective Practice (C. Johns and D. Freshwater, 1998), 133–134
Tournier, Paul
and the person, 8
Trust and boundary violations, 87–90. *See also* Professional malpractice; Professions and professionalism
clinics for treatment, 88, 89
educational resources, 89
and sexual misconduct, 87, 88, 89
The twentieth century
violence in, 15, 35–38

U

Universe, the. *See also* Caring universe; Technology; Teilhard de Chardin; Thomas Berry
and care, 13–14, 41–42
domination and control of, 105–106
and early peoples, 104
as evil, 105
in modern Western culture, 104–105
story of, 101–103, 103–111
study of. *See* Elliot Allen Institute
survival of, 13, 21–22
The Universe Story (T. Berry and B. Swimme, 1992), 103

V

Values
Christian, 118–119
global, 120
Vanier, Jean, 25
Vietnam War
caring in, 32–33
Violence. *See also* The twentieth century
and the absence of care, 30
in the human experience, 27–28, 34
Virtue ethics. *See also* Caring and professional ethics; Ethical discernment; Ethics
and caring, 71, 130
derived from the Greek, 71, 130
differing opinions about, 73
Volunteerism, 25-26
the American paradox of. *See* Robert Wuthnow
and caring, 25–26
in the United States, 25–26
versus altruism, 26, 27
von Hildebrand, Dietrich. *See also* Affective response; *The New Tower of Babel*
and caring as responsivity, 125–127, 128–129
and religio, 108, 109

W

Wagner, Lynn
  and reflective practice, 134
Watson, Jean, 123, 124
Western philosophy. *See* A. MacIntyre
Winter, Gibson
  and the artistic relational paradigm, 121–122
Workplace
  impact on caring, 34
  inability to care in, 90
  and moral ambiguity in, 94
Workplace structures in health care, 90–93. *See also* E. Freidson; Workplace
  bureaucratic labor market in, 91
  controlled labor market in, 91–92
  denominational identity in, 93
  free labor market in, 91
  professional model in, 92
  rational-legal labor market, 91
  secularism in, 93
Wuthnow, Robert
  on volunteerism in the United States, 25–26

X

Xenodochia (houses for strangers), 120